Nurses' Aids Series

PSYCHIATRIC NURSING

THE NURSES' AIDS SERIES

PSYCHIATRIC NURSING

A. ALTSCHUL

B.A.(LOND.), M.Sc.(Edin.), S.R.N., R.M.N.
*Lecturer, Department of Nursing Studies, University of Edinburgh
Formerly Principal Tutor, the Bethlem Royal Hospital and the
Maudsley Hospital, London. Formerly Examiner to the General
Nursing Council for England and Wales*

WITH A FOREWORD BY

D. L. DAVIES

M.A., D.M., D.P.M.
*Physician, Bethlem Royal and Maudsley Hospitals, London
Formerly Dean, Institute of Psychiatry, University of London*

Third Edition

LONDON
BAILLIÈRE, TINDALL AND CASSELL

First Edition April 1957
Reprinted November 1970

Second Edition February 1964
Reprinted June 1966

Third Edition March 1969
Reprinted May 1971

© 1969 BAILLIÈRE, TINDALL AND CASSELL LTD
7 & 8 Henrietta Street, London, W.C.2

SBN 7020 0282 8 Limp edition

SBN 7020 0289 4 Case edition

Published in the United States by the
Williams & Wilkins Company, Baltimore

MADE AND PRINTED OFFSET LITHO IN GREAT BRITAIN BY
COX & WYMAN LTD, LONDON, FAKENHAM AND READING

FOREWORD

IT is five years since the appearance of the last edition of this work, which has been widely received as a valuable and authoritative text. This period has seen the rapid development of certain psychological techniques of treatment, such as behaviour therapy, a bewildering use of new drugs, and an increasing provision of treatment for those addicted to alcohol and other agents, as well as for those whose difficult behaviour is attributable to personality disorders.

In the long term, what may prove to be the most important problem occupying our attention over this period is that of the function of the psychiatric nurse, the setting in which she should work, the pattern of ward organisation, and, necessarily, the kind of training which will best fit her for these.

Where these two elements come together, the changing type of patient and the changing type of nurse (as happens in wards now being set aside for addicts and those with personality disorders), it is true to say that the very survival of such units depends on nothing so much as the attitudes of the nursing staff.

This new edition is therefore well timed, and most welcome in setting out the issues objectively, and in language free from unnecessary jargon. Together with its well established sections on other topics, it should prove a sure guide through an idealogical forest abounding with false trails.

D. L. DAVIES

PREFACE TO THE THIRD EDITION

THIS book is intended to cover the various aspects of psychiatric nursing which every student nurse will need to learn during her training. The syllabus for the examination for admission to the part of the Register for Mental Nurses contains many subjects in addition to psychiatric nursing, since a knowledge of basic sciences, of personal and communal health and of basic bedside nursing is essential for all nurses. The psychiatric nurse must also have a sound knowledge of the causes, the signs and the symptoms of mental disorders, and an understanding of the motivation of human behaviour and of the legal and administrative aspects of her work. Some acquaintance with the manifestations of the more common bodily disorders and with various nursing procedures which she may be expected to carry out is also required.

Since the first edition of this book was published, steady progress has been made in psychiatric care, though nothing has influenced psychiatric treatment as spectacularly as the introduction of tranquillizing drugs in the years preceding the publication of the book. The variety of new drugs continues to be overwhelming and no attempt has been made to deal in detail with the use of specific drugs; only a general discussion of the use of drugs and the dangers associated with them is included. It has been considered desirable to include a short chapter on the care of patients who are dependent on drugs or alcohol.

In this third edition minor alterations have been made in most chapters. In explaining the general principles underlying psychiatric care a threefold approach is outlined: emphasis can be placed on physical treatment, on social aspects of treatment, or on a psychological approach.

Physical treatments, other than the administration of drugs, have fallen into disuse in many hospitals but enquiries show that some psychiatrists continue to rely on physical methods of treatment. The chapters on physical treatment have therefore been abbreviated considerably.

In many psychiatric hospitals great efforts have been made in recent years to develop the community aspects of care and in some hospitals something approaching a therapeutic community has been achieved. Nurses have increasingly taken part in group meetings, conducted discussion groups with patients and developed skills in encouraging group activities. Chapters dealing with this aspect of nursing have been enlarged and there is a new chapter dealing with behaviour therapy. A therapeutic use of nurse-patient relationships is the nurse's special contribution to psychological forms of treatment. Although this aspect of the nurse's work is stressed in every chapter it has been decided to revise the chapters dealing specifically with this subject and summarizing what has been said elsewhere. There are now two separate chapters dealing with relationships and with nurse-patient interactions respectively.

No details of the Mental Health Act can be given in a book of this kind. The brief appendix of notes on the Act is intended only to assist nurses to understand the main principles of the new legislation.

This is a book on psychiatric nursing, not a textbook of psychiatry. It is hoped that the student can understand the patients and the principles of psychiatric nursing without reference to diagnostic categories of mental disorder. The chapters describing the main forms of mental disorder form the last part of the book and should be used only in conjunction with a more comprehensive textbook of psychiatry. Psychiatric nursing is the nursing of people, not of diseases. A good psychiatric nurse must study each patient and think of him as a unique individual who is in need of help. I have endeavoured to indicate how a nurse can help her patients in some of the difficulties which arise in mental illness, and in doing so I have restricted the use of technical language to the essential minimum. The psychiatric nurse's greatest asset is knowing people and knowing about people. To acquire this knowledge she must meet people, talk to them and listen to them. She can also increase her knowledge by reading widely, avidly and critically. Each new acquaintance and each new book will lead to a widening of interest and deeper understanding of human nature. A short list of books which the nurse may find helpful is appended to each chapter.

I have been much heartened by the interest the psychiatric profession has taken in this book and I should like to record my gratitude to all the people who have assisted me in the task of revising the text with criticisms and suggestions. I am indebted to the Editor of the Royal Medico-Psychological Association's *Handbook for Psychiatric Nurses* for permission to use extracts from their glossary.

A. ALTSCHUL

DEPARTMENT OF NURSING STUDIES
UNIVERSITY OF EDINBURGH
December 1968

CONTENTS

PART I

GENERAL PRINCIPLES OF PSYCHIATRIC NURSING

xi

PART II

SPECIAL FORMS OF TREATMENT

PART I

GENERAL PRINCIPLES OF PSYCHIATRIC NURSING

CHAPTER 1

Mental Health and Mental Illness

PSYCHIATRIC nursing is concerned with the promotion of mental health, the prevention of mental disorder and the nursing care of patients who suffer from mental disorder. Psychiatric nurses should know something about the disorders they are helping to prevent and cure, and about mental health which they are trying to restore.

Most textbooks of medicine and nursing begin with a description of the normal and proceed later to describe the abnormal conditions which arise in sickness. Originally, however, knowledge of what is normal and healthy in body and mind was nearly always gained by studying what was abnormal and diseased. Knowledge of the normal functioning of endocrine glands, for example, was discovered as a result of studying abnormalities associated with over- or under-production of hormones. Normal functioning of the brain becomes clearer as more and more is known about patients suffering from brain lesions.

Mental health, too, which has been defined by the World Health Organization, as 'the full and harmonious functioning of the whole personality', can best be studied by reference to mental disorder. If the nurse is seeking to promote the mental health and happiness of her patients, she needs to know what to regard as healthy and what signs to interpret as evidence of disease. As she becomes acquainted with abnormal behaviour she will develop a clear idea of the standards by which she can judge the behaviour of these patients, and of what to regard as normal.

THE DEFINITION OF NORMALITY

What is meant by normality? What does normal life entail?

It is often said that we are all 'a bit abnormal'. Is this true or is it obvious nonsense? Is it any easier if the word 'normal' is replaced by 'healthy', or is it normal to be a little unhealthy?

The difficulty which arises in answering these questions lies in the fact that the word 'normal' is used in more than one sense. It is sometimes employed for 'average' or 'most usual'. By 'normal height' is usually meant 'within certain limits around the average'. But the word 'normal' is not used in this sense when health is being discussed. For instance, it may be found that by a certain age most people have lost their teeth and are wearing dentures, but it is not therefore 'normal' to wear dentures by the age of, say, fifty.

It is often preferred to consider 'normal' as being 'ideal' or 'best possible'. An individual would be called 'normal' in respect of physical health if his organs were functioning in the ideal manner, and 'ill-health' or 'abnormality' are the terms that would be used if there were any serious deviation from the optimal function.

Any particular characteristic or clinical symptom may thus be abnormal when judged by absolute standards, but normal when judged by population standards or vice versa. Outstandingly high intelligence, for example, may approach normality in the sense of 'optimal', but it represents considerable deviation from the 'norm' by population standards.

Deviation from the population norm is not always morbid, as the example of exceptionally high intelligence shows. In old age it may be that a person formerly of outstandingly high intelligence declines to a level approaching the norm for the population as a whole. He then suffers from a disorder characterized by deviation of intelligence from his personal norm.

How about mental health? Here it is difficult to define the ideal without reference to society. It could be said that a person is healthy if he manages to deal with the demands made upon him by society in a manner which is ideal both for society and for himself. He is ill to the degree that he has failed in his adjustment, to the detriment either of society or of himself.

The Normal Adult

What is involved in the life of a normal adult must now be considered. First, it means the normal care of his body. An adult person attends to his personal hygiene in such a manner that he does not come into conflict with society. He washes regularly, attends to his hair, teeth and nails. He is clothed in a manner which conforms to the standards of the society in which he lives. His clothes are reasonably clean, in a reasonable state of repair. They are frequently changed and laundered. The fashions he wears approximate to the accepted styles. He does not walk in the nude, unless in private or in the presence of people who, he knows, do not object. He wears one style of clothes for funerals, another for weddings, and yet others for town or country.

It does not occur to the normal person that there is anything very difficult about this. He does not reflect how much learning was required for the simple achievement of washing and dressing appropriately. Yet there was a time in everybody's life when these actions were not habits. Every child learns by a slow and careful process to wash, and to do so without being reminded. Many people reach adolescence before they are encouraged to decide for themselves what clothes to wear and when to change them. They almost certainly reach adolescence before they buy their own clothes.

Personal hygiene not only involves skills in clothing and washing, but also in elimination. Western society demands that this should be done in private, and convention lays down the right place and time. Conversation about the subject is determined by convention and others may be offended by a too open discussion of bodily functions in words other than those approved by society. This too has been learned during a long, painful apprenticeship, starting in infancy and completed some time during school years. Failure to maintain normal adult standards of personal hygiene is one of the characteristics of some mentally disordered persons.

Normal adults usually take a normal, healthy diet. They do so in spite of certain difficulties they may encounter. They consider meals as being social occasions, pleasurable because of the relief of hunger and the enjoyment of both food and company. They eat regularly, with moderation, and observe a vast number of rules or social conventions. Any mother knows how much effort on her part has gone into the education of her children in this respect. She is justifiably proud when one of her offspring has gone through a whole meal in the presence of visitors without disgracing her. It would be unreasonable to expect a small child to use a knife and fork, to eat tidily, or to refrain from putting his fingers into his mouth. It is often unreasonable to expect it from mentally ill patients.

THE ACTIVITIES OF NORMAL LIFE

Normal life, amongst other things, involves, broadly speaking, the following activities:

(1) adaptation to the work situation;
(2) leisure-time activities;

(3) management of social contacts;
(4) adjustment to the opposite sex.

Each of these headings includes a variety of highly complex activities.

Working, for instance, consists partly in choosing the right kind of job, one which is within reach of the individual's ability, yet making some demands on him. It involves doing the job well and persevering in the face of difficulties. It involves attending the place of work at regular hours, in spite of possible disinclination to do so. At work, other people are encountered—those in authority, colleagues and subordinates. All kinds of complex skills are required in order to adapt to these in all situations.

Work represents the contribution which each person makes to the well-being of society as a whole. Many people find enjoyment in work which is interesting and well done, but many find discipline irksome. For the sake of the community as a whole, work must be carried out at a specified time, and some jobs which must be carried out may be intrinsically unattractive. For some people problems related to work present the main difficulty.

Many people use their leisure time for the pursuits they most enjoy and which make their life richer and more worth while. Leisure is often all too short for the variety of interests people may wish to pursue: art, music, drama, gardening or sports—to name but a few of the many possible and desirable leisure-time activities which may be carried on alone or in company with others. These are often felt to give real purpose to life when work fails to do so. In mental illness failure to find satisfaction in leisure activities is very common.

Making social contacts can be fraught with complications, a fact which becomes plain when consideration is given to the variety of possible relationships and the multitude of adaptations required. Thus, individuals behave in different ways towards their best friends, their neighbours, their clients, their greengrocers. It is difficult to learn the right kind of approach to each, and all embody many possibilities of failure.

Normal adults are continually making new social contacts and discarding others, but there are some friends who remain constant. Real friendship is a mutual relationship. It requires active support from both partners. It is easy to see why some patients appear friendless and lonely, and easy therefore to discern some of the ways in which they may be helped to take up their place in society again.

Normal adults have learned to adjust to the opposite sex. Normal sexual development is fundamental to mental health. Love, companionship and sexual relationships in adult life depend on the social influences which are brought to bear on the sexual development of the child. Many people find sexual adjustment the most difficult task to master.

A brief reminder of what normal life entails should make it easier to understand 'mental illness' and to see clearly the task of the psychiatric nurse. Mental illness can be regarded as a failure to make a satisfactory adaptation to the demands of society.

By taking a history it may be possible to find out why a patient has failed to develop in a normal manner. Heredity, early childhood influences, education, dramatic childhood experiences, may all have contributed to his difficulty. Recent stresses may have caused him to break down at this particular time of his life. His previous personality structure may affect the particular areas of difficulty which he encounters in his adaptation to society.

What are called the symptoms of the disorder are often manifestations of faulty adaptation. Some patients have difficulties in managing the care of their bodies and maintenance of physical health. They require help with dressing, washing, eating and elimination. Others have difficulties in adapting to working conditions, or in finding interest in any leisure activity whatever. Some fail to make friends, and these find social intercourse a burden rather than a source of satisfaction. To many patients sexual adjustment is the greatest source of worry and anxiety, because the standards of society are at the same time rigid and yet ill defined. Whatever the patient's difficulties, they can be thought of as resulting at least partly from excessive demands made by the environment.

Psychiatric treatment involves, in the first instance, simplifying the environmental demands so that the patient can successfully meet them. Often it is possible to do so without admission to hospital. When hospitalization has become necessary the nurse helps to create in the hospital ward a normal, yet simple, flexible routine, adjusted to the patient's needs. Gradually he is helped to learn how to deal successfully with increasingly difficult situations. He is constantly encouraged to tackle more complex problems under the watchful eye of those who are ready to offer a helping hand should it be required. If he encounters failure he is protected from its consequences and encouraged to try again.

Having achieved success in adaptation to hospital life, the patient is helped to meet the requirements of the world at large and to lead a full and satisfying existence.

Books for Further Reading

N. Roberts. (1967) *Mental Health and Mental Illness*. Routledge & Kegan Paul, London.

F. Kräupl Taylor. (1966) *Psychopathology: Its Causes and Symptoms*. Butterworth, London.

D. Russell Davis. (1966) *An Introduction to Psychopathology*. Oxford University Press, London.

CHAPTER 2

The Mentally Ill and the Community

NEARLY half the hospital beds in this country are
occupied by mentally ill or mentally subnormal patients.
Nurses learn in hospital the art of caring for these
patients and of contributing to their recovery and rehabilitation. Most nurses continue to work in hospitals
after completing their training, because in the hospital
team their function is most clearly defined and their
service possibly of greatest use.

Later chapters will describe the way in which hospital
treatment can be of value to the mentally sick patient.
But not all people who require psychiatric help are
admitted to hospital. It would be impossible to provide
accommodation and staff for all. Many derive more
benefit from other forms of treatment.

Although psychiatric nurses at present play only a
small part in the community care of the mentally sick,
they should know something of the social problems of
mental disorder and understand how current attitudes
have developed. Only the barest outline of this can be
given in this chapter. Psychiatric nursing has only a
short history. Traditionally, nurses look after the sick
and helpless, and the concept of mental disorder as
sickness is a very recent one.

HISTORICAL ATTITUDES TO MENTAL DISORDERS

Until the end of the last century, with isolated exceptions, those who suffered from mental disorder were ignored or ridiculed, unless they were obviously dangerous to the community. Those who were thought to be dangerous were, at various periods, executed, illtreated or imprisoned. They were considered as being totally different from other human beings, chained and kept under physical restraint, physically and mentally tortured in order to render them manageable.

Pinel in France (1745–1826), and Tuke in York (1732–1822), proclaimed that the insane person was human, and would respond to kindness. Pinel, watched by a frightened and disbelieving audience, removed the chains and convinced his followers that the time was ripe for humane treatment of the insane. Education was required, both of those who were responsible for the care of the insane, and of society as a whole, before some of the fear of the insane person was lost, and sufficient sympathy and interest acquired to abandon restraint. In 1891 the first course of instruction was given to attendants of the insane in this country.

As public opinion changed, so people became less disposed to hide their affliction, and it became clear how large was the number of people who would benefit by humane care. Lunatic asylums were built where many thousands took refuge from an unsympathetic world too difficult for them to understand.

Not until the end of the nineteenth century was the public conscience sufficiently aroused in England to accept, by Act of Parliament, official responsibility for the care of the insane, to delegate this duty to local authorities, and at the same time to admit that the person of unsound mind required the protection of the law from those who might be sufficiently unscrupulous to take advantage of their afflictions.

The Lunacy Act of 1890 clearly laid down the circumstances in which society had the right to protect itself from those who might cause damage as a result of mental disorder. It defined the responsibility of the local authority to provide care and protection, free of charge, for those who were certified to be in need of it, and it laid down in detail the extent to which a person deprived of his liberty by virtue of certification was entitled to protection and to the safeguard of many of the rights of citizenship.

As time passed, many of the safeguards against wrongful certification, exploitation and ill-treatment appeared no longer to be necessary. Better staff was employed in mental hospitals, and public opinion had moved towards sympathy and understanding.

While wrongful certification became an unlikely occurrence, fear of mental illness and the stigma associated with it prevented maintenance of interest in the patient after certification. Feelings of fear, shame and guilt caused relatives to delay certification as long as possible but, once this had become necessary, quickly to forget the patient. The situation of many asylums made visiting difficult, and there was a tendency to think of admission to an asylum as final. Many asylums, with their large, beautiful grounds, became self-contained communities, a refuge for patients from the harsh world outside.

Modern Attitude to Mental Disorders

While public opinion gradually moved to an acceptance of responsibility for the humane care of the mentally disturbed, expert opinion approached the recognition of mental disorder as an illness requiring medical and nursing care. Medical interest was devoted to careful description of abnormal behaviour, in an attempt to classify and diagnose it, and to prescribe treatment. Psychiatric nurses were needed in place of attendants for the insane. The new function of the nurse consisted in accurate recordings of signs and symptoms, and in helping to detect early manifestations of mental disorder with a view to treatment and prevention.

Fear of certification, however, mitigated against early treatment of mental disorder, and a new method for the admission of patients became necessary. In 1930 the Mental Treatment Act made it possible to receive treatment in a mental hospital as a voluntary or temporary patient, without legal formalities, and yet retain the protection granted to certified patients. The Mental Treatment Act was preceded by a similar Act in Scotland, and in England by a special Act of Parliament granting the London County Council permission to treat voluntary patients at Maudsley Hospital.

To emphasize the recognition of mental disorder as illness the name 'asylum' was changed to 'mental hospital', the word 'patient' substituted for 'lunatic', and 'nurse' for 'attendant'.

As the attitude of the public towards the mentally ill became increasingly sympathetic and understanding, many people became aware that the legislation relating to mental disorder was still unnecessarily complex and restrictive. In particular, concern was expressed about the fact that many people detained in institutions for the mentally defective did not appear to be discharged as readily as seemed to be desirable. A Royal Commission was set up in 1954 to enquire into the way the law was operating and to make recommendations for change. As a result of it, the Mental Health Act was passed in 1959 and the Mental Health (Scotland) Act in 1960. They came into operation in 1961.

The essence of the Act is reflected in its title. *Mental health* rather than disease is the subject of the Act. All previous legislation relating to mental illness and to mental deficiency is now obsolete and the aim of the new Act is to abolish all distinction between the way people suffering from physical and mental disorder are treated.

The term *mental disorder* was introduced to cover all psychiatric conditions. For the purpose of the Act these disorders are classified into:

(1) Mental Illness
(2) Mental Subnormality
(3) Severe Mental Subnormality
(4) Psychopathic Disorders

The Act abolishes Mental Hospitals as specially designated hospitals. All patients now have the opportunity of being admitted to any hospital able to offer them treatment. All hospitals may offer treatment to any patient they feel they can help and may refuse to admit patients whom they do not feel able to help. Clearly, many hospitals continue to specialize in certain types of treatment and many psychiatric patients require specialized care, but there is no legal restriction on other hospitals or patients.

Most patients suffering from 'mental disorder' are admitted to hospital in precisely the same manner as if they were suffering from any other kind of illness. A few patients only require to be admitted or detained against their will. Medical certificates from two doctors are sufficient to ensure that patients receive the treatment they need. In Scotland such an application for admission has to be approved by the sheriff. Patients who feel that they are wrongfully detailed have, however, recourse to specially constituted Mental Health Review Tribunals or, in Scotland, to the Mental Welfare Commission.

Investigations into the causes and treatment of mental illness developed along divergent lines. On the one hand, the chance discovery of malarial therapy for the treatment of general paralysis of the insane led to a search for organic causes and physical treatment. On the other hand, the findings of Freud and his followers led to increased understanding of personality development and the factors causing faulty adjustment. Investigation of psychological and social causes of mental disorder and treatment by psychotherapy and social influences made rapid strides.

The general interest in the prevention of illness which has yielded such marked results in other fields of medicine has spread to psychiatry. There is a belief that there must be a right and a wrong way of bringing up children, that more knowledge of the psychopathology of mental disorder would lead to clearer understanding of how mental disorder can be prevented. Anxiety and unhappiness, not previously recognized as mental disorders, are now seen to be relevant, and there is a widening interest in child care and in the social and educational responsibility for developing healthy mental attitudes.

COMMUNITY CARE

Since the orbit of mental disorder has widened to include neuroses and social maladjustment, hospital care is no longer considered to be the best form of treatment for all. At present there is a growing awareness of the responsibility of the community as a whole for the rehabilitation of those who have suffered. Many people believe that hospitalization should be resorted to only if no other method of treatment is possible. Removal of the patient from his own environment makes it unnecessarily difficult for him to return to it when he has improved. Treatment of the patient in his own setting is considered to be preferable whenever this is possible. Many general practitioners have become alerted to the high incidence of mental disorder in the population and are treating their patients effectively with or without consultation of a psychiatrist.

Closer contact between the patient's own doctor and the psychiatric specialists seems desirable. Some psychiatrists consider domiciliary visits to the patient to be the most effective way of persuading him to agree to have treatment. Psychiatric out-patient departments in many general hospitals provide necessary treatments without interfering with the patient's adjustment at home. If more intensive therapy is required, 'day hospitals' provide all the therapeutic resources of in-patient treatment, without the disruptive effect of removal from home and admission to hospital. Day hospital treatment avoids the complete removal of responsibility from the patient and spares him the effort of readjusting to his environment on discharge.

If community care of psychiatric patients becomes the method of choice for most patients, more help will have to be available to relatives. More psychiatric social workers will be required to give help and support to the patient's family, and to understand their problems and difficulties. Education of the general public towards greater tolerance of the mentally ill is still necessary.

Many psychiatric patients are able to carry on only in a relatively sheltered atmosphere. Some kinds of hostels may be required where those who do not need hospital care can nevertheless receive some measure of shelter and protection. Many psychiatric patients are able to work well and efficiently provided they do not have to work in competition with normal people. Special forms of sheltered employment may be required where, in spite of their disablement, mentally ill people can earn an independent living, and benefit from the increased self-respect which is supplied by gainful employment.

TRENDS IN PSYCHIATRIC CARE

The present trend of psychiatric care is summarized below.

.There is an increased awareness of the responsibility of the community to the mentally ill. On the whole, there is a tendency to keep patients out of psychiatric hospitals, or to return them to the community as quickly as possible. Within the community greater understanding of the needs of the mentally ill is being developed, and also a greater awareness of the social causes of maladjustment.

Within the hospital there are three main trends of thought, which are as follows:

(1) There is a growing amount of information available about physiological disturbance in mental patients, accompanied by an increasing use of physical methods of treatment, especially drugs.

(2) There is an interest in the psychological causation of faulty attitudes, an exploration of unconscious goals and motives. Psychotherapeutic techniques are developing along various lines.

(3) The significance of social factors in the causation and treatment of mental illness is recognized. The interaction of patient groups is being studied, the effect of staff on patients is better understood, and the hospital in many instances is developing into a therapeutic community.

General principles of care are the same whether the patient receives treatment in hospital or in the community. Whatever the causes or manifestation of the patient's illness, some failure in adjustment to the demands of society always occurs. Therefore, in order to help the patient, some attempt must be made to adjust society to the patient in the first instance. Wherever possible this should happen within the patient's own community. His friends, relatives, employer, might, with the help of the psychiatric team and as a result of changed attitudes, adapt to the patient. Where this is not possible, the patient needs treatment in the special environment of a psychiatric ward, be it in a day centre, in a general hospital or in a psychiatric hospital.

The aim of treatment is, however, to help the patient to learn new methods of adjustment. The phase during which the environment adapts to the patient should not be unnecessarily prolonged, nor should the demands made on the patient be excessively reduced. Everything that is healthy should be preserved; wherever the patient is capable of acting in a normal, healthy, independent manner he should have an opportunity to do so.

The patient may need help to improve his physical condition or, on the other hand, he may be physically fit and well and need only the opportunity to maintain his usual state of nutrition, exercise and physical care. He may have a reduced capacity to work, earn his living and assume responsibility for his dependants, and treatment may have to include help in this respect. On the other hand, the patient may be quite competent in all that is involved in working and should not, during treatment, be allowed to lose his skill or his sense of responsibility.

If the patient does not require active assistance in making friends or in using his leisure time he should not, during illness, be allowed to lose his social skills, his interests or his circle of friends. If he does have difficulty, the hospital should offer the patient the opportunity to learn how to form new and more satisfying friendship patterns.

Community care offers the best opportunity for retaining all that is best in the patient's adjustment. Hospital care in what is described as a therapeutic community may be necessary where the patient needs to learn or re-learn social living.

BOOKS FOR FURTHER READING

H. Freeman (Ed.). (1965) *Psychiatric Hospital Care*. Baillière, Tindall & Cassell, London.

H. L. Freeman & J. Farndale (Eds.). (1963) *Trends in Mental Health Services*. Pergamon Press, Oxford.

A. Strauss and Others. (1964) *Psychiatric Ideologies and Institutions*. Free Press of Glencoe, Collier-Macmillan, London.

CHAPTER 3

Therapeutic Environment

FOR those who require in-patient treatment, the psychiatric hospital provides not only nursing and medical care but, temporarily, also a home and security. The patient's treatment begins from the moment of admission into the therapeutic surroundings of the hospital.

Most patients, before admission, have lived through a period of tension and strain. The patient may have realized his increasing inability to adjust to the demands made by society, and after desperate attempts to cope may have broken down suddenly under the stress, or may gradually have understood the need for treatment.

The patient's family may also have been exposed to considerable strain. Often, as a patient's symptoms develop, he is subjected to comment, criticism and reproach. Gradually, as it becomes clear that he is ill and unable to control his behaviour, the relatives become worried and anxious. They watch suspiciously for further proof of insanity and consequently the patient becomes more irritable and tense. Eventually, as the need for the patient's admission to hospital becomes obvious, the relatives feel guilty and partially responsible for his breakdown, ashamed and emotionally disturbed.

The patient's arrival in hospital may mark the climax of an intensely disturbed home situation. The feeling of guilt, added to misconceptions about psychiatric hospitals, may have led the family to delay as long as possible the patient's admission. The actual removal to hospital is sometimes an unpleasant procedure, force may have to be used, or considerable effort expended in persuading the patient to enter hospital. In almost every case, admission to a psychiatric hospital represents a crisis in the patient's life and that of his family. In any crisis people are more able and willing to accept help if it is offered than they would at any other time. The way patients and their relatives are received into hospital is therefore a significant aspect of treatment.

The hospital must provide the environment suitable for the patient's needs. His illness makes it impossible for him to adapt himself to his environment, therefore in hospital the environment is adapted to the patient. Outside, he has reacted to specific stress by becoming ill; in hospital, stress can be removed or controlled so that the patient can learn to deal with it.

The psychiatric hospital must be able to adapt to all kinds of patients—the most helpless and those who have almost recovered, the most antisocial or withdrawn and the most excited and active. Each patient from the moment of admission should feel that the hospital can provide security and the kind of atmosphere in which recovery is possible.

Several factors combine to create the therapeutic atmosphere of the hospital:

(a) the structure and arrangement of the ward;
(b) the attitude of the staff;
(c) the morale of the ward community as a whole.

The Structure and Arrangement of the Wards

Most patients are pleasantly surprised to find that wards look more like home than hospital. In all wards the aim should be to create an atmosphere of warmth, comfort and relaxation. Colour, tastefully decorated rooms, attention to the arrangement of furniture, pictures, flowers, help to give the ward a homely atmosphere. Cleanliness and order are necessary, but should not deprive the patients of comfort.

It is often the practice to arrange each ward differently, in a way suitable for one group of patients only, graded as to the amount of difficulty presented to the patient who moves from ward to ward as he improves or as his symptoms become worse.

This is not, however, the only way in which accommodation in hospital can be utilized. Some believe that it is beneficial for the patient to remain in one ward throughout his stay. This allows time for him to get to know the staff really well, and to form sound, enduring relationships with nurses and with other patients. It helps him to feel secure, because he knows that, whatever his behaviour, he will not be transferred and that the people looking after him are capable of helping. As he improves he can take an increasingly active part in caring for others and assuming responsibility for himself.

Where the opinion prevails that it is in the best interest of the patient to remain in one ward throughout his stay, the patient's age rather than the mental disorder determines to which ward he is admitted. Where the hospital is very small or where there is a single psychiatric ward in a general hospital, it is inevitable that patients remain in one ward throughout their stay.

There are some advantages, however, in thinking of the hospital as a total community able to accommodate patients in different wards according to their need for protection or their ability, or otherwise, to act more independently. The patients readily see that the move to a more unrestricted environment represents progress and improvement.

Careful preparation is necessary to ensure that transfer from one ward to another proves to be therapeutic. The patient needs to prepare himself for the move, plan how to collect his belongings, inform his visitors and take leave from the patients with whom he shared a ward. A little party or other celebration may be a suitable way to mark the occasion. He may wish to become acquainted with the staff and patients of his new ward before the move is actually made and he may wish to retain some contact with the staff and patients of the ward he is leaving by promising frequent return visits.

Unfortunately, while it is beneficial to the patient to feel he is progressing when he moves to a ward offering more scope and responsibility, it is distressing for him to be aware of a relapse when a move in the reverse direction is necessary. It requires considerable skill to convey to the patient that different wards are neither better nor worse, but just more suitable to help patients at specific stages of illness.

Size of Wards

The size of wards is of significance in the treatment of the patient.

While he is very ill, helpless or disturbed, he benefits from a small ward where he is exposed to only a few people and where it is easy to comprehend the physical layout. The patient may derive a considerable feeling of security from the knowledge that he is physically safe and always accompanied by a dependable person whom he knows well.

As the patient improves, the space he occupies can be enlarged. Bedroom, dayroom, dining-room, kitchen and bathrooms become accessible to him. Within the precincts of the ward and ward garden the patient may be free to explore. He makes his own decisions as to where he spends his time. He is more exposed to contact with other patients, and has an opportunity of trying to establish friendships, assuming leadership or making other social relationships.

Before the patient is discharged to his home, he requires yet more complex surroundings. Far from being shut in, the patient should have full opportunity to move freely within the hospital and in the neighbourhood. He should use his own discretion about going out on pass.

In order to cater for all patients the psychiatric hospital should be large enough to have all the facilities required in a community, but not so large that the patient feels out of touch with part of his environment. Hospitals of 100 to 300 beds have been found of greatest benefit. There should be suitable wards for patients of all kinds. Ground floor wards should be provided for the old and infirm who need direct access from ward to garden. Small, sheltered, enclosed gardens should be available for those who are disturbed; large grounds and sports facilities should exist for those who can benefit from exercise. There should be workshops catering for all needs, work available from the simplest to the most complex types, with working conditions as near normal as possible for those about to be discharged, but able also to give the most sheltered employment to those who need it.

A community centre is required, a large entertainment hall for special occasions, smaller rooms for more informal social occasions, rooms for organized gatherings and rooms where men and women can mix in an informal manner. Library, reading-rooms, shop and canteen can be most valuable additions to hospital amenities.

Before discharge the patient's environment should be widened to include the local community, traffic and contact with people outside. The patient can then lead a full life organized by himself. He meets plenty of people and relies on his own initiative in associating with them. Facilities for hobbies and entertainments are provided, but it is left to the patient to decide how they are used. He should feel responsible for the care of the wards and be invited to interest himself in the welfare of others and to make suggestions for the running of the hospital. In short, the hospital is a training ground, albeit a safer one than the outside world, for life in the community.

ATTITUDE OF STAFF

In order to make the best possible use of the facilities of the hospital the nurses need to understand fully the aim of treatment and the reasons why the hospital is used in the way it is. The patients' attitude to treatment may well depend on the attitude conveyed by nurses.

In some hospitals the ward for the most disturbed patients is kept locked. This is distressing to many patients though a few patients feel more secure and protected in a closed ward.

The hospital's responsibility towards the community and for the safety of helpless and potentially dangerous patients must be recognized. Many psychiatrists and nurses believe that they can fulfil their responsibilities without resorting to the locking of doors. Increased skill in observation, a greater degree of patient participation in the management of the ward and a programme of active occupational therapy help them to give adequate attention to those patients who are known to be in danger of wandering away or who might behave dangerously if they were permitted to leave.

Others believe, however, that the security of locked doors permits the nursing staff to give all their attention to active treatment rather than to custodial care.

If the ward is locked patients may become extremely disturbed. Excitement, anger and possibly violence may result from the frustrating experience of being locked in; and patients, who might otherwise be quite willing to accept treatment, become determined to leave the ward. Patients may develop resentment towards the nurse who holds the key and even the most unobtrusive handling of keys and the greatest care in preventing noise of locking and unlocking may result in casting the nurse in the role of custodial authority. The nurse's positive attitude is of cardinal importance if the closed ward is to be used therapeutically.

The nurses' attitudes are also of great importance to new patients. Many patients feel extremely apprehensive about entering hospital. Some have heard rumours of ill-treatment, some are afraid that, once in the hospital, they will be there for ever, some simply fear the stigma of the psychiatric hospital and are convinced that their friends and relatives will despise them for having been admitted. Many patients, despite explanations from their doctor, are certain that mental health is simply a matter of willpower, and they despise themselves for having 'given in' instead of 'pulling themselves together'. If the nurses can succeed in creating a happy, warm, hopeful atmosphere, confident, relaxed, yet purposive, patients can soon be convinced that their decision to enter hospital was the right one.

Some patients, on arrival in hospital, are worried by the sight of patients more disturbed than they are themselves. However, the opportunity to observe the kind way in which another patient is being helped by a nurse is often most reassuring. It is important to learn that the nurses can remain calmly in control when other patients become disturbed. It may help the patient to feel sufficient confidence in the staff to risk letting go of his self-control for a while, and this may be a necessary preliminary to successful treatment.

Patients sometimes complain that very little is being done for them in hospital. This is because they fail to understand how the experience of living in a ward which has just the right kind of atmosphere for recovery can be part of 'treatment'. Explanations do little to convince the patient. Even so, it is necessary that the nurses themselves should be clear about the effect of atmosphere and should understand how they themselves are responsible for engendering therapeutic rather than anti-therapeutic attitudes.

Some nurses find it easy to understand patients who are very ill. They can readily maintain a calm and accepting attitude in the face of even the most disturbed behaviour. But when patients begin to improve nurses sometimes become irritable and intolerant.

When a patient is very ill the constraints of firm rules and regular routine are helpful but they become irksome as the patient improves. It is essential that the patient should be enabled to experiment with freedom and responsibility as he gains independence and self-confidence.

These experiments are not always entirely successful and some attempt may have to be made to exert control. But if nurses enforce discipline in an authoritarian manner, the patient's recovery can be very much delayed.

A new patient can feel very bewildered by the many new experiences of admission to the psychiatric hospital. Though he may need to ask many questions, he may feel unable to give voice to any of them, because he feels embarrassed, insecure and unable to know which of the many people he meets could be asked. In some cases the remedy may lie in admitting the patient to a small ward unit where he will find only very few people to whom he can easily be introduced. If the patient goes to bed when he first arrives, he is spared the embarrassment of moving around and introducing himself. Instead, staff and patients approach the patient one by one. If each person who speaks to the patient introduces himself the patient can very quickly be helped to feel that he belongs.

It is, however, emphasizing the patient's dependence and illness if he is asked to go to bed soon after arrival in hospital. In many wards it seems more desirable to emphasize the normal healthy aspects of ward life. This can be done more easily if a patient, rather than a nurse, takes on the role of host and is responsible for introductions, explanations and orientation.

Whatever admission procedure is adopted it must be recognized that every new patient has many unspoken fears and anxieties. The nurses' attitude will either assist the patient to ask, or it will stop all questioning.

Nothing the patient wants to know is too trivial for discussion but the patient cannot always formulate his problems clearly. At the early stage of a patient's stay in hospital answers to his questions may not in fact be known, but that should not prevent the patient from asking.

What is appreciated by patients is a nurse who has time to listen and whose attitude suggests that she would like to know more clearly what is worrying the patient.

Whenever an answer is possible it should be frank and clear. But hasty answers, before questions are fully expressed, merely serve to convince the patient of the futility of asking.

Some patients have heard rumours of ill-treatment, restraint and padded cells. They cannot put into words the question they would like to ask. For example: 'How are these people going to treat me? Are they as kind as they look? Can they be trusted? Are they competent? What will they think of me when they realize how bad I am?' Instead of asking these questions patients may put the nurses to the test; becoming, for example, either mute or hostile and aggressive.

The best way of convincing the patient of his nurse's interest in him is by her being interested. He must be convinced that his abnormal behaviour, which is the reason for his admission to hospital, is considered neither shameful nor wicked. The patient must never be condemned or ridiculed. The non-critical attitude of the staff may help him to relax and so recovery may be hastened. However inappropriate or disturbed the patient's behaviour, he must feel that he is accepted and wanted in the ward.

The nurse should convey to the patient that she considers all the information she obtains from or about him as being strictly confidential. It may be a great relief to patients and relatives that nothing about his illness will be known to anyone, except those concerned with treatment.

Many of the patient's actions during the worst phases of his illness are capable of leading later to the greatest embarrassment. Some of the information which psychiatrists, and sometimes nurses, receive about the patient's private life is divulged with the greatest misgivings. The patient must be able to rely on the integrity of every member of the staff as to the observance of the necessary secrecy.

MORALE OF THE WARD COMMUNITY AS A WHOLE

It is impossible to over-emphasize the importance of harmony amongst all members of the staff. There is no simple way of telling nurses how to get on with each other. A harmonious ward is the result of every individual working to the best of his ability with the interest of the patients at heart. Harmony results from a confidence that all are capable of coping with difficult situations, and that the efforts of one are appreciated by the others. It is the result of mutual confidence and trust. When the staff work in harmony with each other, the patients' behaviour usually presents very few problems, and what nursing problems arise are easily settled.

In every working community friction occasionally arises and usually results from personality clashes. In psychiatric nursing it arises more commonly from differences of opinion about the correct method of nursing the patient, and the latter becomes anxious because it affects him so intimately. Careful observation of the incidence of excitement in disturbed wards has shown very clearly the relationship between patients' anxieties and dis-agreement among staff.

Whenever difficulties arise in the ward it is worth while to examine the attitude of staff members to each other, and to have a free discussion about the way each feels. Exchange of opinion about the correct manner of handling a situation is possible only if each nurse feels secure in her relationships with the others. Inevitably mistakes are sometimes made, often there is an aware-ness of the wrong thing having been said to a patient. These mistakes can be discussed and their repetition avoided only if no nurse feels personally insulted or criticized. Sometimes the feeling of envy at another nurse's success, or of frustration at individual inability to make contact with a patient, may lead to staff tensions.

Some patients create ill-feeling among nurses by playing them off against each other, criticizing one nurse in the presence of another, making each feel that the other gives more attention.

For many patients the continuous support of the nurse represents the first sign of friendship in what appears to be a hostile world. Admission to the hospital may mark the end of a period of loneliness and the beginning of social participation in which the other patients as well as the staff have a vital part to play.

In the opening chapters it has been shown that mental illness can be regarded as some failure in adjustment to social change. Difficulties in work, leisure activities and social contacts with friends and relations represent the main problems with which the psychiatrically ill person has to deal.

Irrespective of the specific diagnosis of a patient, the

aim of treatment is to restore or to enhance the patient's ability to cope with changing circumstances of his life.

The psychiatric hospital provides the training ground within which the patient can learn to form healthier relationships with people and to modify his behaviour.

There are three different approaches to the problems of mental illness:

(1) There is the possibility of using *physical methods* of treatment. Much research is taking place in efforts to discover an organic base for psychiatric disease. So far, this research has met with only very limited success. In a later chapter this will be discussed in more detail. But although there is little evidence of organic cause of most mental disorder, there is increasing interest in the effect of various drugs on the patient's symptoms and behaviour. Treatment by physical methods can therefore be of considerable significance.

(2) Because adult behaviour is the outcome of the complex influences any person experiences during the process of growing up, it is profitable to explore the life history of each patient. Patients' attitudes are frequently indicative of childhood problems, many of which have become unconscious. *Psychotherapy* is a form of treatment in which the connections between present and past in the patient's experience are systematically explored. Diagnosis and treatment overlap because the process of bringing unconscious motives into consciousness helps the patient to understand his difficulties and to choose better adapted behaviour subsequently.

(3) The patient's current problems in social adjustment may be regarded as the most important. The fact that the patient has managed without psychiatric help until the recent past suggests that the insurmountable difficulties are to be found in the precipitating circumstances and the social pressures of the environment from which the patient was admitted. Treatment is concerned primarily with the social factors of the patient's life, with

modification in the demands made on the patient, and with support for the patient while he learns to cope with the problems which arise. This approach to treatment is often referred to as a *socio-therapeutic* one.

The three possible approaches are, of course, interrelated. Success of physical treatment is dependent on the relationship between the patient, the doctor who prescribes it and the nurse who administers it. These relationships are dependent on the patient's earlier experiences and attitudes.

In-patient therapy, even when it is intended to be of physical or psychotherapeutic nature, takes place in the social environment of the ward and the hospital. When that environment is therapeutic the patient's progress is often quite dramatic. When a therapeutic environment is not created patients fail to progress.

The greatest contribution the psychiatric nurse has to offer lies in the ability to create the social climate in which the patient can get well. In the chapters which follow it will be shown how this can be achieved.

Books for Further Reading

J. S. Bockoven. (1963) *Moral Treatment in American Psychiatry*. Springer Publishing Co., New York.

E. Goffman. (1968) *Asylums*. Penguin Books, Harmondsworth, Mddx.

M. Greenblatt, R. H. Y. York and E. L. Brown. (1955) *From Custodial to Therapeutic Care in Mental Hospitals*. Russell Sage Foundation, New York.

World Health Organization Public Health Papers No. 1. (1959) *Psychiatric Services and Architecture* W.H.O., Geneva

CHAPTER 4

Ward Routine

ROUTINE is an important stabilizing factor in life.

It is well known that children become unhappy when their familiar routine is disturbed.

Nurses derive great security from knowing the routine of the ward in which they work and feel disturbed each time they move to another ward, until the new routine is mastered.

Ward routine is important to patients too, and if it is adjusted to the special needs of the patients it plays an important part in therapy.

In order to understand the value of the established routine to any particular patient, the nurse should know something about the life led by patients in their own homes. Some will have led a very well-regulated life prior to admission. They may have been slaves to routine and punctuality may have been the keynote of their lives. Some obsessional patients, for instance, have spent much time and energy arranging time-tables and organizing themselves and others. Difficulties of adhering to the schedules may have been major factors in the development of the illness. While some patients may have always worried about routine, others may never have adhered to any form of time-table. Some patients have never been sufficiently independent to organize their own lives, others have never been sufficiently concerned with the rules of society to consider other people.

Ward routine must therefore be planned according to the patient's individual problems.

1. *Should the routine be simple or complex?*

In some wards only the very simplest sequence of events has any chance of succeeding. Where patients are demented, confused, disorientated, where there are patients who are incontinent or incapable of attending to their personal hygiene, routine should consist almost entirely of meals, toilet, washing, dressing and undressing. Exercise and a certain amount of occupation must be included, but the main purpose of treatment is to teach such patients to care for their own bodily needs and, by adhering very firmly to a routine, gradually to establish socially acceptable habits. A simple routine does not, however, provide adequate opportunity for most patients.

2. *Should the routine be inflexible or is it advisable to allow some variation?*

For some patients it is essential that routine be firmly established. Many have become insecure and anxious because they have failed to keep up with changes in their home circumstances. Some have succeeded in disrupting the home by their illness. The fact that hospital routine is stable, invariable and not dependent on the patient's behaviour may do much to aid recovery. To know that the future is predictable, that it is independent of the patient's own actions, may be most reassuring at some stages of his illness.

It is essential, however, that variation in routine should occur sometimes to avoid boredom.

People have not only a daily routine but also a weekly one and a yearly. If all the days of the week resemble each other, time becomes difficult to measure. It is important that Sunday should be different from weekdays and preferable that each day of the week should be marked by some special event. The weekly menu, or the favourite T.V. programme, or the evening entertainment can help to differentiate between days. Visiting days and shopping days can mark the highlight of the week.

It is part of the yearly routine that one celebrates birthdays, Christmas and Easter, that there are holiday week-ends and a longer break in work when one goes away.

3. *To what extent should the routine be arranged for the patient, and to what extent should the patients be responsible for their own arrangements?*

In some wards, all arrangements must be made by the staff. To the minutest detail everything is prearranged.

A clock and a calendar are of course essential items of ward equipment. Time-tables are made out and posted on the wall. Everybody sees at a glance what they should do at every moment of the day. Work is distributed, a rota made out, nothing left to chance. This may be very helpful for an anxious or obsessional patient, and it may help to rehabilitate some withdrawn schizophrenic patients who would otherwise be inactive, hiding where nobody would pay attention to them. But it would not be a good preparation for resuming responsibilities outside hospital.

So, in other wards, only the bare skeleton of the ward routine is rigid. Meal-times are the usual landmarks. Everything else is left to the patients to arrange. Time-tables may be made out by the patients at meetings, or some patients may be entrusted with a particular section of routine, e.g. the arrangements for ward cleaning, or the organization for serving meals or for entertainments.

In some wards, no formal arrangements are made, division of labour evolves as a natural process and by mutual agreement among patients.

The nurse's role varies considerably in these different

types of routine. She may assume a role of authority, she may become an elected leader, or she may become a member of the group, indistinguishable in function, as far as ward routine is concerned, from the patients themselves. She should know what is expected of her in the ward in which she is working, and she should be able to sustain this part and cope with the anxieties she encounters in those patients who have difficulties in adapting themselves.

Patients move from ward to ward, and sometimes react very strongly the first time they are expected to make their own decisions. They look to the nurse for guidance and become hostile and critical when they do not receive it. This can be anticipated and dealt with by the nurse who properly understands her function. A nurse who does not thoroughly understand this either becomes disturbed about the patients' criticism, or, as a result of her own insecurity, critical of the ward sister. Only frequent discussion of the problems at issue can help the nurse to maintain her proper position.

4. *How important is it that patients should adhere to routine? How much initiative on the part of the patient should be encouraged?*

Every now and then patients who break hospital rules are encountered. They come in late from pass, or they go out without letting anyone know. They are late for meals, or stay in bed longer than others. They decide to stay away from occupations or disapprove of the entertainment organized for them. In short, they rebel. Nurses often become disturbed by this type of behaviour. Their problem is how to persuade the patient to conform, but often they omit to ask whether it is essential for him to do so. Might it not be a good thing if the patient shows a little independence?

It should never be forgotten that the aim and purpose of treatment is not to create docile hospital inmates, but to help patients to deal adequately with an infinite variety of difficulties in life outside the hospital walls. A little experimentation is essential if the patient is to succeed. This does not mean that hospital routine should be discarded, or that persistent breaking of hospital rules should be condoned. The nurse, however, is better equipped to deal with the problem if it is seen as a welcome sign of growing independence. Often the first attempt of a patient to break a rule is merely tentative. He is afraid of the consequences. It would be all too easy to prevent any further show of a growing sense of self-confidence if the first attempt is dealt with tactlessly. All that is required is a willingness to find out why the patient behaved as he did and, instead of showing indignation, try to get the patient to understand why the rule is necessary and why it must be kept.

Among other difficulties the patient must learn to cope with the displeasure of the staff, e.g. the ward sister. It is perfectly all right to show disapproval of an action, provided the patient knows that the nurse is as interested as ever in him and his welfare, that he is liked and valued, in spite of the fact that an individual act could not be permitted. A great deal, however, depends on the way in which the patient is censured, and on its timing. It is essential for nurses to plan what are to be their reactions to the breaking of rules. No two patients require the same approach. Spontaneous anger or indignation is rarely helpful and criticism should be resorted to only when it is known that the patient is well enough to tolerate it. Otherwise a different ward, with different routines, may be necessary for a patient who persistently violates the conventions of the one he is in.

5. *How much time in the routine of the ward should be devoted to each activity?*

The answer to this question is dependent on the age

of the patients and the degree of illness. The sequence of events is on the whole fairly similar in different wards. The patients rise, wash and dress. Then follows breakfast, bedmaking, cleaning of wards, occupation and exercise. After the midday meal there is clearing up to be done. The afternoon is spent in occupation, leisure activities, entertainment, with tea and supper in between. Lastly, there follows evening toilet and bed. These, interspersed with physical treatments and interviews with doctors, are the usual events in a patient's life.

The amount of time devoted to each item should be carefully determined. If patients are old, the speed of activities must be reduced. Plenty of time must be available for each one, changes should be few, and plenty of warning should be given. If many patients require supervision during morning toilet, more time must be allowed for this than is required in a ward where all patients are able to look after themselves, and are soon returning to work. Meals should always be unhurried, but require more time when patients need to be fed and carefully supervised.

In some wards it is essential that some time should be entirely free, and that patients should be encouraged to plan their own leisure. In other wards it is preferable that the whole day should be covered by the ward routine. Nurses should be clear about the amount of help required by their patients. Sometimes it is far better to allow more time, e.g. for ward cleaning, but to give little help; sometimes it may be more desirable to ensure that things are done, even if the nurses themselves have to do a good deal of the work.

The right kind of routine is an essential tool in therapy. The patient cannot be expected to realize this, and it is understandable that patients look for active treatment and often complain that they receive none. If the nurse herself is not clear why things are different in one ward from what they may be in the next, she may find it hard to persuade the patient, who, when he sees things done differently in each ward, is apt to feel that hospital routine is haphazard and purposeless. If the nurse understands the reason for everything that is being done, she is able to deal effectively with the patient's worries and help him greatly by her attitude of confidence and reassurance.

CHAPTER 5

Observation and Reports

OBSERVATION and accurate reporting are amongst the most important functions of the mental nurse.

Psychiatric treatment is the more effective, the more it is based on a thorough knowledge of the patient's personality. Everything he has done in his life and everything that has happened to him have contributed to make him the kind of person he is. The psychiatrist tries to find out as much as he can about the patient by interviewing him and, with the patient's permission, his closest relatives and possibly other people who can give information. He obtains further details from the psychiatric social worker. He forms a picture of the patient's mental state, and supplements his own impression with the results of psychological tests.

Additional information is supplied by the nurse, who gives a picture of the patient as he appears in the ward setting, and an account of his behaviour from day to day.

Accurate and objective observation and reporting must be learnt. Observation of all details is impossible; what is noticed and interpreted as being significant depends upon the nurse's experience and knowledge. It is impossible to report every detail of every event, but training enables the nurse to select the most relevant and significant particulars for her reports.

Because all observation is selective and determined by the observer's 'set', i.e. his expectation, attention, knowlege and preoccupations, it is valuable to compare reports from several people. In hospital it is possible to make use of the observations of a number of nurses, to pay particular attention to those observations which are borne out by others, and to investigate the reasons for conflicting observations and reports.

THE BASIC PRINCIPLES OF OBSERVATION

The following are some of the basic principles which must be followed if the best results are to be obtained.

The nurse should know what information she is seeking. One can only notice what is significant if observation is accompanied by knowledge.

1. A knowledge of normal behaviour pattern in different cultural groups is essential. What is accepted as normal behaviour differs with social class, with different educational background, and with nationality. It is important to observe to what extent the patient's behaviour deviates from that accepted by his own group. Without a background knowledge of sociology there is danger that the nurse's own social class and educational background may bias her observations. Where nurses and patients come from different countries, particularly if they do not share a language, special care is needed to make observation valid.

2. The nurse should be acquainted with the possible patterns of abnormal behaviour and their incidence in various mental disorders. A knowledge of psychology and of psychiatric illness may help to detect the earliest manifestations of disorder, when these may well be atypical and different in each patient. Many disturbances can be avoided if nurses become sensitive to the earliest signs of anxiety in the patients.

3. The nurse should be with the patient for sufficient time to be able to report on the total picture he presents.

Only if she knows him intimately can she observe minor variations in behaviour.

4. The nurse must not disturb the patient by her presence. This means that she must be in the ward so much that her presence is taken for granted and that she is sufficiently unobtrusive for patients to behave as if she were not there at all. She can best observe the individual patient's behaviour if she joins in all the activities. If she comes and goes she disturbs these and cannot obtain a true picture of individual behaviour. If she supervises passively, doing nothing while the patient is expected to take part in some ward activity, her presence may be resented and the impression she gains then becomes distorted.

5. The nurse should be an objective observer. For this reason she must not allow herself to become neither very disturbed or frightened by the patient's behaviour, nor shocked and angry. Her interest in his recovery should not make her emotionally biased. She must not feel flattered at, or proud of, his improvement, since this might lead her to see improvements where there are none. One of the reasons why relatives are sometimes unreliable informants is their inability to remain emotionally detached. Close emotional contact with the patient may be desirable but it interferes with objective observation.

6. The nurse should remember to observe the total situation in which the patient finds himself. To do this is relatively easy when the nurse's report concerns the interaction between several patients, or that between the patient and another nurse. It is much more difficult if the nurse is reporting an incident in which she herself has been concerned. The patient's behaviour which she observes is then a reaction to her own words, actions or gestures. It may require considerable mental effort to report such behaviour not as it appeared to her, but as she imagines it might have appeared to a third person.

Her own part in the interaction needs to be reported as well as the patient's.

7. Although it is impossible to observe the patient's behaviour without to some extent interpreting or making guesses about underlying motives and forming judgments about his personality, it is absolutely essential that observed facts should be reported, and not merely opinions; or at least that, when opinions are given, these should provide some indication of the facts on which they are based.

Good Reporting

Clichés should as far as possible be avoided. Such words as 'pleasant and co-operative' mean nothing unless it is stated who finds the patient pleasant and for what reason, and what were the tasks in which the patient was expected to co-operate. 'Unco-operative', again, describes the relationship between the patient and someone else. It is important to know with whom he refused to co-operate, and what attempts were made to persuade him to do so.

Some expressions, such as 'bizarre behaviour' or 'incoherent speech', are meaningful to a certain extent, because they are used by most people to apply to the same kinds of phenomena. Nevertheless definite examples are better than the mere statement that the nurse failed to understand the patient.

There should be some plan for carrying out and recording observations, in order to ensure that no significant aspects of the patient's behaviour are missed and that the total picture of this becomes available rather than one distorted by the high-lighting of episodes. There are many useful ways of arranging observations in categories under a variety of headings. One possible method is to consider all the various situations covered in a twenty-four hour period, and to list the activities in which observations can be made. More detailed discussion of the nursing problems associated with these observations follows in Chapters 7 to 11.

OPPORTUNITIES FOR OBSERVATION

At Night

The nurse is in a position to observe the patient in bed. The manner of his sleep is a very important clue to diagnosis. He may settle down early or feel more lively in the evening. He may sleep well in the first part of the night, but wake up before the other patients, sleep lightly or deeply, wake frequently, or lie awake for long hours. He may be calm in spite of insomnia or may be worried and anxious at night. During the first few days in hospital the patient's reactions to sleeping in a dormitory should be recorded and his attitude to being under observation at night.

Physical Health

Personal appearance and appetite can sometimes be used as a guide to the patient's physical health. Any changes, such as pallor or flushed skin, pained facial expression, difficulty in walking, should be noted. Changes in the amount of interest the patient takes in his appearance or his meals should be carefully investigated.

Toilet

In the morning, the nurse observes the patient's manner of dressing. She notices whether or not he is careful of his appearance, how long he takes to wash, whether he is meticulously careful in his toilet, or quick and superficial. The training which the patient has had as a child, his usual standards of dress and grooming may be revealed as well as the degree to which his present behaviour is disturbed.

Meals

Meal-times offer an opportunity to observe the patient's table manners, to discuss his likes and dislikes as regards food, and possibly to obtain some inkling of his attitude to his family with regard to food standards. He may compare hospital food with that cooked by his wife and talk about her qualities or shortcomings as a cook. He may reveal whether he expects the lion's share at home, or whether he cares if his wife and family are well fed. Sometimes, if financial worries play a part in the patient's problems, or have done so in the past, discussion about food may lead to suggestions made by the patient on possible remedies.

Work

The patient's attitude to work is another important field of observation. Consideration here should be given to how much work he is able to do, whether he starts working spontaneously or needs persuasion; whether he is energetic or listless; keen, interested, eager to learn new things, or timid and reluctant to try new ideas. His punctuality in starting a task and his perseverance in difficult situations are of importance, and so also are the questions of whether he can stand up to correction, whether he aims at a very high standard or is content with slipshod work, whether he prefers to work alone, or likes to work in company. The nurse can notice if he is a leader or a follower in the group and whether he prefers to work by himself or with someone else.

Leisure Activities

Nothing is more revealing than observations about leisure activities, interests and hobbies. It is of importance to know if the patient likes dancing or goes only because all the others go. His interest in the week's entertainment programme, whether he talks about it in advance, persuades others to take an interest, or is aloof and apathetic, should all be given observation. The nurse will know the patient better if she is acquainted with the kinds of entertainments he dislikes or criticizes and those which appeal to him.

It is interesting to know what books the patient reads, how fast he reads, what strikes him as beautiful or as being worthy of discussion. Sometimes it is useful to read the same books as some of the patients in order to have a common topic of conversation. Newspapers should always be read, since these frequently form the basis for communication.

Visitors

It is most important to observe the patient's reactions to visitors or to receiving letters. The patient may give much information about his friends or family to a nurse whom he considers to be interested and sympathetic. His behaviour may change following a visit from a particular person, or he may become excited whenever he expects a visit from his wife. Some patients, although eagerly looking forward to a visit all the week, are abusive to visitors when they come. The responses of the patient to the mother, husband or boy friend may throw some light on the psychopathology of the illness. The relatives' reactions to the patient may be even more revealing and so might be the patient's disappointment if no visitors arrive.

The patient's behaviour on being admitted to hospital, his attitude to staff and other patients, to hospital life and hospital rules are points of significance. Later his approach to newly admitted patients, to unusual incidents in the ward, to a change of nursing staff, to transfer to another ward, are all matters of interest. Christmas festivities, sports day, the annual dance, a coach outing, may provide opportunities for observing hitherto unknown facts.

Obtaining Information

The nurse obtains information about the patient, not by asking questions but in an indirect way. She first establishes rapport with him by showing that she is interested and a willing listener. She must be interested in anything he chooses to tell her and in everything he does. The first approach is usually a trivial one. The patient wants to know which nurse, if any, he can talk to and approaches all nurses with some little story or some unimportant remark. Only when he becomes convinced that the nurse feels interested in him and that she does not laugh at or criticize him, does he continue to single her out and give her an opportunity of learning more about him. Every conversation she has with the patient, no matter what the topic, gives some indication as to his life, general upbringing and past experiences. Every time the nurse observes the patient, alone or in a group, at rest or at some activity, she acquires more information about his personality. Her task of convincing him of her real interest in him is the easier, the more topics of common interest she can find. In order to sustain conversations the nurse should have as wide a knowledge and as many interests as possible. She can increase her knowledge considerably by listening to patients who talk about their jobs, their hobbies or their opinions.

It is never the nurse's function to argue with the patient, or to expound her own opinions on controversial matters such as politics or religion. To show interest in the patient's point of view is valuable, not to convert the patient to one's own.

Reports

Reports about patients are given verbally and in writing, for a variety of purposes, and must therefore take a number of different forms. Day and night reports are usually written for administrative purposes. They are not intended to give a picture of the patient's mental state or progress. They are designed to indicate to the next shift some of the treatments carried out, dramatic changes which have taken place and events which may be of significance.

Nursing administrators should be able to discover from these reports, if possible at a glance, whether the ward is adequately staffed, taking into consideration any special events which have occurred. They should be able to redistribute nursing staff or take any other action considered desirable in the light of the reports.

Reports should mention all the patients in the ward, state how many and which of them are on the danger list, bedfast or having treatment for physical illness. They should indicate those patients who require special observation because of suicidal thoughts or because of excitement or violence. Patients who require tube feeding or who are incontinent are usually mentioned because of the demand made on the nurses' time. Patients who are away from the ward, at occupations or out on pass are listed because their absence from the ward reduces the nurses' work. New patients are mentioned and their condition briefly described. Transfers and deaths are reported. Attention is drawn to other administrative details.

These reports are written in all hospitals with the full knowledge of the patients. They are necessary for the efficient administration of the ward, but they do not usually give any helpful information to the patient's doctor. Often a Kardex system is used as the simplest method of record keeping.

Confidential Information

Where there is close co-operation and team-work between doctors, nurses and other workers much more detailed information about the patient must be exchanged. All aspects of his behaviour may be reported and discussed. Interchange of information is essential for effective teamwork. There are however, important ethical problems which must be considered. Frequently the patients are unaware that such reporting takes place. Much of the information given to the doctor or to a particular nurse may be considered confidential by the patient and he would be reluctant to speak if he were aware of the interchange of observations. If he specifically states that he wishes information to remain confidential the doctor may feel obliged to withhold it from the nurse, or may decide to give the necessary instructions verbally, rather than to make the notes about the patient available to the nursing staff

Before the nurse obtains confidential information from the patient, she should try to persuade him to discuss the matter with the doctor. But if the patient does not wish to do so the nurse must make it quite clear to the doctor that she is passing on information against the patient's wish. Preferably it should then be given verbally to the doctor, rather than committed to paper. No nurse or doctor should ever use in conversation knowledge obtained from a third person. The doctor can try in an interview to obtain directly from the patient, information to which the nurse has drawn attention.

If the doctor gives the nurse some details about the patient's history, for example the fact that the patient has deserted his wife, the nurse can learn from this information to avoid the subject or can try to win over the patient to tell her about his marital problems, but she cannot talk about it to the patient until he chooses to tell her.

Progress notes written about patients can take various forms.

They can be tabulated under a number of headings, as, for instance, the following:

Appearance
Speech
Appetite
Sleep
Interests
Occupation
Attitude to staff
Attitude to other patients
Attitude to visitors

They may also be written in essay form, in which case the nurse is free to omit some aspects of the patient's behaviour and enlarge on others which appear to her to be significant.

Whatever the method, care should be taken to give an over-all picture of the patient's behaviour, not only to high-light specific incidents. Over a period of time the reports should give a clear picture of his progress.

As each nurse spends only 42 hours per week on duty and only a small part of this time in the company of any one patient, it is inevitable that several nurses should be concerned in the observation of every patient.

It is often helpful if a nurse can take a special interest and feel responsible for collecting information about her patient from all her colleagues. This ensures that all nurses have an opportunity of sharing knowledge with each other, of expressing opinions and avoiding misunderstandings. It ensures that reporting is comprehensive and that a coherent picture is presented.

CHAPTER 6

Problems of Physical Illness in Psychiatric Patients

THE OBSERVATION OF SYMPTOMS

AMONGST psychiatric patients, as in any large group of people, there is always some incidence of physical illness and the nurse must deal with it as she would in any other hospital. Some problems, however, are peculiar to psychiatric hospitals and require particular skill and conscientiousness on the nurse's part, and special consideration in determining ward routine. These problems may be summarized as follows:

(1) Many mentally ill patients may be physically ill without complaining.

(2) Some mentally ill patients complain almost constantly of their physical symptoms, and this may be an indication of their mental rather than their physical state; yet sometimes these patients are in fact physically ill also.

(3) Infectious illness is liable to spread rapidly in psychiatric hospitals.

Care of patients who do not complain

In order to discover physical illness at the earliest possible moment and deal with it effectively, in spite of the fact that the nurse cannot always expect very much help from the patients, she must be extremely observant. If she knows her patient really well she can note the slightest deviation from his usual state.

A thorough knowledge of the signs and symptoms of the most commonly occurring physical diseases is necessary. Knowing what combination of symptoms to expect helps to detect early the presence of physical illness.

The nurse should always know about the possible ill-effect of any drugs she is administering and watch for complications.

The ward routine is designed to help in discovering early signs of physical illness. It is rare to take the temperature, pulse and respiration of every patient as a matter of routine in mental hospitals and therefore much depends on the nurse's own powers of observation. There are, however, some other routine procedures which are helpful.

Every patient has a very thorough physical examination on admission and not less than once yearly throughout his stay in hospital. He has regular dental examinations and treatment, and in some hospitals regular chest X-rays. Blood tests may be done as routine on admission to detect patients suffering from syphilis and to detect the effects of any drugs patients may have been in the habit of taking. Bromides and amphetamine are detected in this way. Early stages of diabetes mellitus can be discovered as a result of routine urine testing.

It is helpful if the nurse, on the patient's admission, writes a brief description of him which will enable anyone seeing him some months later to estimate whether he looks better, worse, or about the same. Patients are weighed at regular intervals, and excessive increase in weight, or loss of weight, is investigated. Excessive weight may indicate endocrine disorder, increase in weight may be due to oedema. Loss of weight may indicate such disorders as tuberculosis, thyrotoxicosis, or may be due to insufficient food intake or excessive energy output.

Sometimes it is necessary that the patient's body be inspected when he has a bath. Any scars, bruises or deformities are recorded in writing, so that any fresh mark on his body can be immediately recognized as being new.

With women patients a record should be kept of menstrual periods. Examination of the patient's clothing may be necessary. Amenorrhoea should be noticed and the reasons found; these vary according to age. Amenorrhoea frequently occurs in psychotic patients and may be no indication of organic disorder. On the other hand it may herald pulmonary tuberculosis or endocrine disturbances. Pregnancy, as a cause of amenorrhoea, should not be overlooked. Abnormal or irregular vaginal discharge should be noted. Where so many patients are elderly, it is most important to discover early signs of malignant growth or of fibroid tumours, which might lead to serious haemorrhage. Some patients conceal objects in the vagina and may either injure themselves or cause infection and a purulent discharge.

Some attempt should be made by the nurse to keep informed about the patient's bowel actions and micturition. She should notice if a patient goes to the lavatory frequently. Some patients need to be asked if they have had their bowels open, but sometimes it is necessary to accompany patients to the lavatory. It is then possible to see if the patient is constipated or has diarrhoea, if he appears to be in pain on micturition, if he passes large or small amounts of urine, or if he has frequency of micturition. Specimens of urine should be tested at regular intervals if there is any reason to suspect urinary disorder.

Meals are supervised and loss of appetite, apparent discomfort or pain on eating, abnormal craving for any particular type of food or excessive thirst should be reported and investigated. Nausea and vomiting require instant attention.

One of the most difficult symptoms to observe is pain,

if the patient does not trouble to refer to it. It is necessary to know the patient very well indeed in order to make accurate observations. He may have a limp, or walk with difficulty, find it an effort to rise or sit down, have difficulty in swallowing. His facial expression may reveal pain. He may frequently touch a part of his body; for instance, his forehead. He may be quieter, less lively than usual, sometimes more amenable and less disturbed. All these changes may indicate pain. Questions may then elicit details. The patient may be unable to answer if he is asked, 'Are you in pain?' but reply readily if asked, 'Where is your pain?' If the patient is flushed or pale, excessively quiet or behaves in a manner unusual for him, he should be examined and put to bed, until the nature of his illness is clear.

Care of patients who frequently complain

The patient who frequently complains of physical malaise is difficult to nurse. Anxious patients often complain of palpitations, difficulty in breathing, nausea, headaches and many other symptoms. Hysterical patients may describe symptoms which suggest every conceivable physical illness. Nearly always, in such cases, physical investigations have been exhaustively carried out before admission to a psychiatric hospital. In the absence of organic findings the patients may have been diagnosed as 'neurotic'. The pains are real and serve a purpose. The patient requires treatment, not for his symptoms, but for the underlying illness, which makes it necessary for him to have these physical symptoms. The doctor, having carefully examined the patient, takes great trouble and time to explain that there is nothing physically wrong and that worry, anxiety and emotional upheavals may cause very real physical sufferings. Treating physical symptoms by drugs or surgery will not help the patient but will serve only to convince him that, after all, there is something physically wrong.

This presents, however, a very real problem to the nurse if some physical illness develops in addition to the patient's neurosis. The patient may not, as he supposes, have heart disease, but he may suffer from an attack of pneumonia. He may not have anything wrong with his stomach but he can develop appendicitis; he may not have a paralysed leg, but he can sprain his ankle. How to differentiate between organic illness when it arises and neurotic or psychosomatic symptoms, how to give adequate attention to the patient's physical symptom without appearing to take too much notice of the symptomatic manifestations of the neurosis, is impossible to describe. It may be enough to be aware of the problem for all the nurses to pool their information about a patient and together plan how to observe unobtrusively the signs and symptoms he presents.

There are many symptoms which may first be observed by the nurse. Dehydration, a very dangerous symptom which may have many causes and lead to serious effects, should be discovered by the nurse who supervises the patient's toilet and attends to his oral hygiene. It often accompanies enteric infection. What looks like sunburn may be the first sign of pellagra. Slurred speech may be due to some neurological condition, or to the sore tongue of vitamin deficiency. A patient who resents all attempts to persuade him to go into the garden for exercise may have fractured his leg or suffer from a septic toe. Only incessant vigilance and personal interest in patients can bring about early diagnosis of their physical illnesses.

PREVENTION OF THE SPREAD OF INFECTION

It is frequently reported that the incidence of certain infectious illnesses, e.g. enteric infections and tuberculosis, is high in psychiatric hospitals. There has in recent years been an outbreak of smallpox in a psychiatric hospital. Patients who do not complain could cause serious spread of these infections before the disease is diagnosed. It is essential therefore that those suffering from infectious diseases should be isolated at the earliest possible moment, and early diagnosis is of paramount importance.

When an epidemic of enteric infection occurs, it is sometimes advisable to take specimens of stools from all contacts, or to obtain rectal smears, which is much simpler.

To detect tuberculosis, sputum may have to be sent to the laboratory. Since many patients are incapable of giving specimens, or may swallow their sputum, gastric washings may have to be obtained for analysis. Examination of clothing for evidence of faecal incontinence or diarrhoea is important in enteric infections and so is the examination of handkerchiefs or the provision of rags or paper tissues for patients who cough.

The nursing of patients with infectious illness can create major problems, first because the facilities for adequate isolation cannot always be found, and second, because nurses cannot always count on the patient's co-operation. It is the nurse's function to keep the patient isolated in bed to prevent the mixing up of fomites, i.e. articles which have been used by or have been in contact with the infected patient, and to attend to all the precautions to which other patients would normally attend. In the case of a tuberculous patient it may require ingenuity to prevent the patient spitting or soiling his fingers with sputum.

Even if the sick person is adequately nursed, the prevention of spread cannot be assured unless the problem is tackled along 'public health' lines. Just as in a village community search would be made for the cause of the illness, carriers traced, contacts isolated and general steps taken to prevent spread, so, in a psychiatric hospital, the problem must be dealt with systematically.

In the community the incidence of infectious illness drops if living conditions improve. Living conditions in the ward should be raised to the highest possible level. To increase their resistance to disease, patients must be adequately nourished and have plenty of fresh air and exercise. Food should be well cooked and served, nourishing, well balanced and appetizing and each patient must have an adequate diet. Exercise in the open air should be made so enjoyable that the patients look forward to it, and have healthier appetites as a result of exercise.

Overcrowding always contributes to the spread of disease. Psychiatric hospital wards are often overcrowded, especially sleeping quarters. The nurse should bear this in mind when an infection is being traced and should arrange for examination of those patients who sleep near one who has an infectious illness. Placing the beds head to foot may help. During the day, overcrowding can to a certain extent be overcome by using a wide area for a variety of activities which take place simultaneously. Whenever possible, patients should be away from the ward during the day. Lavatory and washing facilities should be adequate for the number of patients and the nurse must see that they are properly used and kept clean.

When an epidemic has occurred, all the services of the hospital should be checked in order to make sure that no possible way of spread is left open. The water supply and sewage disposal system are usually adequate but it is as well to have these examined by the engineers. The waste water pipes in washrooms and bathrooms often run into a gully before running outside the building. This may be useful when dealing with patients who might try to dispose of some of their belongings down the drain, but it may also be an added source of danger. The food supply is a likely source of infection because patients often work in kitchens, bakeries and butcher's shop and may cause contamination. Patients also work in store-rooms and on farms. Only those who are absolutely healthy should be allowed to do work of such a kind. The laundry and linen rooms must be inspected because careless laundering of infected clothing may easily lead to further spread.

The factors which cannot be over-emphasized are:

(1) the education of patients and staff, and
(2) the supervision of patients

All patients should be aware of the importance of washing hands after each visit to the lavatory and the nurses should see to it that enough time is allowed for this. Soap and towels must be supplied and toilet supervised. The patient's clothing should be clean, frequently changed, adequately laundered. The nurse should ensure that each patient has clean clothes and should see that clothing is neatly put away at night, preferably in separate lockers. Scrupulous attention to food hygiene is essential and only those patients should be allowed to work in kitchens who can be taught the elements of personal hygiene. It is possible by using skill and patience, and by good example, to teach even the most deteriorated patients to look after themselves. Co-operation is required from those patients who could be a source of widespread infection and every member of the staff should aim at standards of health and cleanliness comparable at least with those of the community at large.

CHAPTER 7

Personal Hygiene

MOST people spend a considerable amount of time, energy and thought on the care of their own persons. They try to buy clothes which fit well, look nice and are made of good and lasting material. They dress as well as their financial situation permits and devote great care to their clothes. Much time is spent washing and ironing; clothes are hung or folded carefully in order not to crease them and to keep them in good condition.

Some people are much interested in the washing, ironing and cleaning of clothes. Others find this is a drudgery which they would gladly delegate if they could.

Personal hygiene, bathing, washing, care of hair and nails and elimination present few problems to normal healthy people. Few reflect on how much effort it has cost their parents to teach them the value of cleanliness, the habit of washing and shaving, the right time and place for defæcation. This highly organized aspect of behaviour has become habit and is carried out almost automatically. In sickness the individual becomes aware of the complexity of these details of daily occurrence.

Nurses who care for those who are physically ill devote a great deal of their time and skill to the personal hygiene of their patients. They learn early in their training how to wash and bathe patients in bed and in the bathroom, how and why to care for the mouths of helpless patients, how to give urinals and bedpans.

The mental nurse needs to learn all these things and, in addition, she must learn why some of her patients do not appear to care for cleanliness, why others want to wash all day long; why some patients do not bother to make themselves attractive and others take so long over dressing that they would never reach the breakfast table if they were not helped. She must learn how to persuade the patient to wash or to stop washing, and she must try to understand why one nurse is sometimes successful in persuading a patient to undress, while another may dismally fail to do so.

Attention to the patient's personal hygiene calls for skill and understanding and offers unique opportunity for establishing rapport with him, for obtaining valuable information and for helping him in a personal way.

Most patients are quite capable of looking after their own bodies and their own clothing. All that is required is adequate washing facilities, sufficient time, sufficient privacy and enough cupboard space for clothes. Most patients have regular baths, cut their nails if a pair of scissors is available, wash their hair, go to the lavatory, change their underwear quite regularly without prompting. In order to be sure that the patient is not neglecting any aspect of personal hygiene, it is the routine in most hospitals that a nurse is present in the bathroom at least on some occasions. The nurse uses this opportunity for observing the patient, noticing any scars, bruises, rashes or other abnormalities. Tact is required to help the patient overcome the embarrassment of having a nurse present.

Bathing is a pleasant activity. The patient should enjoy his bath, it should not be hurried. The patient should have a chance to relax and enjoy the pleasant sensation of hot water. Most people like to lie in the bath for a while. Many people sing or whistle in the bath. Patients often begin to talk. The intimacy of this situation can be most valuable. At times, the bathroom is the only place where the patient feels sufficiently relaxed to speak, and he may then sometimes confide to the nurse problems he would not have braced himself to mention in any other situation. It is most important that the pleasure and the intimacy of the bathing situation should not be ruined by hurry or by having several patients in the bathroom at once.

Given the opportunity, men usually shave regularly because they feel uncomfortable when unshaven. Each man is the best judge of the frequency with which he needs to shave. Electric razors may safely be used without the need for supervision.

Shaving is usually supervised when razor blades are used. In the hands of suicidal patients they can be very dangerous indeed. In some wards razors are given out by nurses and collected again after use. Some patients must be shaved by the nurse. All this is time-consuming and shaving should be carried out only when enough staff is available and when there is no danger of nurses being diverted to other tasks and relaxing vigilance.

Regular haircuts for men and attention to hair styles in women are most important. Some hospitals have hairdressing shops, but, failing this, a keen and enthusiastic nursing staff can work wonders with the patients' hair. Patients may be enabled to try out new styles on each other and keen interest in hairdressing may then develop. The use of cosmetics is always encouraged and a few complimentary remarks from a nurse, a doctor or another patient may give back to the patient some of the self-respect that may have been lost.

Clothes

Whenever possible patients wear their own clothes. These fit well and patients have good reason to look after them. Facilities for washing and ironing or for sending clothes to the laundry should be provided. Dress sense can be encouraged by the nurse if patients are helped to dress suitably for various occasions, differently for work, for dancing or for going out shopping. Mirrors must of course be freely available. Women need at least one full-length mirror in order to ensure that they are well dressed.

Clothes assume considerable significance in most people's lives. Tastes differ and the way people dress is often characteristic of their personality. When looking at clothes in a shop window or admiring another person's dress, one tends to imagine the clothes on oneself. 'This dress would suit me', or 'This colour is not for me', are expressions which indicate that people's ideas of themselves often include their clothes. Their concept of their own identity is closely connected with the clothes they wear. Some people feel as acutely upset if their clothes suffer damage as if their own body were involved.

Because clothes are so intimately bound up with body image and feeling of identity, it is important that patients should have the opportunity of dressing as well and as distinctively as possible. Adequate time for good grooming is essential and patients benefit if they can choose their own clothes, go out personally to buy clothes or, sometimes, make their own dresses. Washing, ironing, dry cleaning, mending and altering clothes may take up a fair amount of the patients' time and a good deal of their interest.

When patients have been in hospital for a long time it may be difficult for them to know how much clothes cost and they may need help in planning how to save money and how to budget in order to buy a specific item of wardrobe. Some patients suffering from schizophrenia have particularly marked difficulty in assessing their own identity. They often have problems with their body image. For these patients, it is particularly important that they should possess their own clothing and that they should dress in their own distinctive manner.

Elimination

Most patients go to the lavatory regularly, but the nurse should know if the patient passes urine normally and has his bowels open daily. She should observe any abnormality, e.g. frequent visits to the lavatory, and show enough interest to encourage the patient to report any abnormality he himself notices.

Some patients need assistance in their personal hygiene at the time of the menstrual period. Behaviour changes often accompany menstruation.

DIFFICULT PATIENTS

So far, consideration has been given to patients who require no more from the nurse than interest, encouragement and adequate bathroom facilities. There are, however, many others who need a great deal more than this. At one extreme there are patients who, left to themselves, are incontinent of urine and faeces, who defaecate and urinate wherever they stand. Some patients play with faeces, smear it on walls or eat it. There are patients who would remain in the nude if they were allowed to do so. There are patients whose hair becomes matted, who would never wash unaided, never change their clothes of their own accord. Some of these are patients in schizophrenic stupor or in extreme excitement. Some manic patients are so restless, preoccupied and excited that they have no time to wash or dress. The tongue becomes dry and cracked, the skin sore. Clothes irritate them, they prefer to be naked. Some depressed patients simply have not the energy to wash or change their clothes. They are unable to make the effort to go to the lavatory. Some schizophrenic patients gradually lose interest in their appearance. They spend more and more time alone in their rooms and finally become neglected. Demented patients, those who have an organic brain disorder, e.g. those with general paralysis of the insane, often pass through a phase of completely degraded behaviour. They may neglect their own health and appearance. They sometimes use articles for purposes for which they are not intended. They may use the toothbrush for shoe cleaning, or use someone else's flannel. They often soil their clothing, and if not watched may hide dirty underwear in quite unexpected places.

All these patients require very careful and skilled nursing, if their health is not to suffer. They render themselves liable to infection and they also increase many times the danger of spreading infection should this occur. Their care may take up the major part of the day in some wards. Habit training, of which more will be said later, very largely consists in re-establishing habits of washing, dressing and attending to the toilet automatically, without having to think or be reminded. On the part of the nurse, vigilance is needed, perseverance and scrupulous punctuality, as well as encouragement of the slightest effort on the part of the patient.

Some patients refuse to dress. Some may hear voices telling them to undress, or may feel unworthy of the clothes they are wearing. Others believe that they are poor, that nothing, not even their clothing, belongs to them. Some patients think that their clothes are germ-infested or that they smell. A patient may refuse to be dressed by a particular nurse because he thinks she is his enemy. He may fear that if he dresses he will be led away by the police. No amount of coaxing or persuasion can be successful unless the specific reason for refusal to dress is known and the patient can be convinced of the nurse's understanding. The patient may become very angry with the nurse who tries to make him dress against his wish, but he may submit if she indicates that she takes the responsibility for any consequences which the patient fears may result. It may, however, be necessary to wait until the patient's mood has changed, or until a nurse trusted by him is available.

INCONTINENT PATIENTS

Incontinence and neglect of personal appearance occur quite commonly in the withdrawn patient and should be recognized as an indication of the degree of the patient's illness. His behaviour should not arouse strong emotional reaction in the nurse, and the patient should be protected also from the expressed disapproval of the group of fellow patients who may feel disgust at, or intolerance of, his disregard of social standards.

On the other hand, it may be equally wrong to accept incontinence as inevitable and to become resigned to its occurrence. Incontinence is sometimes a significant activity, a manner of communicating on a non-verbal level, something which is meaningful to the patient, but difficult to understand. The patient's incontinence may follow a regular pattern, it may occur only if he is alone, or always when a certain nurse is on duty. It may be a means of gaining attention or a manner of protesting against an action the patient may not wish to perform. One patient's incontinence may occur only in the ward, never in the garden, another patient may void urine each time the doctor passes through the ward without speaking to him.

It may be very rewarding to discover if there is any recognizable meaning in the patient's incontinence and to prevent its occurrence by giving him personal interest.

It is extremely embarrassing for the patient to be incontinent. Everything possible should be done to save the patient this embarrassment. In many instances incontinence diminishes if the patient is up and dressed. Patients who are confined to bed have great difficulties attracting the attention of a nurse in time to obtain a bedpan or a commode. It is also easier to detect the restlessness which precedes micturition, and which accompanies constipation, if the patient is up than when he is in bed.

Some patients are incontinent simply because the lavatory is so far away that it is difficult for them to reach it in time, and confused patients may have difficulty in finding their way there.

Attention to the patient's toilet is the most personal service a nurse can give him. By giving it willingly, if possible anticipating his need, she can do more than she can by any other method to convince him of her interest.

OBSESSIONAL PATIENTS

One of the most difficult problems with which the nurse may have to deal is that of managing patients who insist on washing over and over again. Obsessional patients may wash many times a day, or may take so long over their morning toilet that they find it difficult to arrive at breakfast. In the evening, hours are spent in folding shirts. Every time the patient goes to the lavatory or touches a door handle he again washes his hands.

If these patients are stopped, they become intensely unhappy and anxious. If allowed to carry on, they occupy the bathroom all day, prevent others from using it and are quite incapacitated for other activities. When dealing with patients of this type, personal hygiene may become a matter of secondary importance. With the doctor's help a plan must be drawn up, to say whether the patient is to be allowed to carry on his compulsive actions or whether the risk is to be taken of making him more anxious by interference.

It is important to try to understand what an obsession may mean to the patient. Water may have a symbolic significance, handwashing may perhaps be symbolic for the washing away of guilt. The doctor may be able to discover the reason for the patient's guilt feeling. If the latter's behaviour has some special meaning for him he cannot give it up unless he can solve his unconscious conflicts. Once the nurse's curiosity is aroused and she is interested in why the patient behaves in the way he does, she ceases to be anxious about routine and has thus taken the first step in helping the patient, to whom her interest and willingness to understand is of great value.

CHAPTER 8

The Significance of Food

___

FOOD AND SOCIETY

IN order to appreciate the problems mental nurses may encounter in relation to food, consideration must first be given to the importance of food in the lives of most people. Fortunately, extreme hunger is rare in Western civilization and it is difficult to realize how powerful a motive the hunger drive can be. In concentration camps, or in countries in which part of the population is literally starving, the importance of food and drink in human life can be only too tragically observed. Normal human beings, given the material means, provide themselves with an adequate, well-balanced diet. Their behaviour, their social and ethical standards, their cultural achievements, are determined by factors other than the hunger drive. Because hunger is so rare in Western society, the actions of other drives, e.g. that of sex, can be observed in a more uninhibited way, and this may be the reason why some writers have attributed to it a disproportionate importance.

But even in a society which is rarely hungry, food plays an extremely important part. Political issues are decided on such problems as food prices and food production. Revolutions have begun over the price of bread or the dumping of grain into the sea. International treaties are formed and broken according to the nutritional needs of nations, and wars are won or lost by the maintenance or otherwise of a food supply line.

FOOD IN THE HOME

Individual lives centre around food. Housewives spend a large proportion of their time planning meals, buying, preparing and cooking food. Marital relationships may be influenced by the quality of the wife's cooking. Meals form central pivots for people's activity. Meal-times are relatively fixed landmarks in the day, and people tend to make them the central points of their lives. Friends are entertained to dinner, restaurants are visited when others are casually encountered. Evening outings begin or end with a meal. Business deals are closed over luncheons, successes are celebrated with food and drink. It is necessary only to observe the engagements of such a person as the mayor of a city in order to see how important is food in public life. Food, apart from its social significance, has great psychological importance.

FOOD AND THE CHILD

Sucking is one of the baby's first activities, his first contact with the mother. Milk is the baby's first source of satisfaction. If infant feeding is properly managed the mother who provides milk soon becomes the object of the child's love. The mother first holds and cuddles her child during feeding and she derives her greatest happiness from this contact.

When the mother withdraws the breast the baby is for the first time deprived of something he needs. Very early the baby loves and hates his mother, according to the satisfaction or frustration experienced in the feeding situation. The first conflict in the baby's life arises. If breast feeding is difficult both mother and child become anxious and derive little satisfaction. Many feeding problems may arise early in life. Parents worry about and discuss the relative value of breast feeding versus bottle feeding, of scheduled feeding versus feeding on demand.

They cope with weaning problems, they have to battle with food fads, with refusal of food or with excessive eating in their children. Table manners are taught and the child gradually learns to acquire the tastes of its elders.

If the child grows up in a warm, secure family setting, if it is loved and gains approval for its achievements, it succeeds in learning the complex skills related to adult enjoyment of food. If, however, the child is hampered in its development, some of its difficulties are expressed at meal-times.

Refusal of food is a very powerful weapon, arousing intense emotion in the parents. The mother may become excessively concerned about the child's health and, because of this, give him more affection and attention. She may become angry about his obstinate refusal of food. In the scenes that follow the child asserts his strength, but everybody becomes unhappy and disturbed. Meals, instead of being pleasurable occasions, are dreaded by all because of the uncomfortable atmosphere created by the child. The unhappy child loses its appetite and feeding problems are intensified.

Later in life individual attitudes to food very largely depend on early experiences and associations. Some people, when they are worried and unhappy, feel sick and lose appetite. Others find in food their only solace. Food may always remain symbolic for love. The offer of a meal by one person to another may be an indication of the relationship between them.

FOOD AND THE PATIENT

In hospital the patient is dependent on others for the satisfaction of all his bodily needs. Nurses are very much aware of the fact that they establish emotional contact with the patient when they offer him food or have to feed him. They realize that the patient's praise of food represents an appreciation of the general care he receives. A great deal of thought is given to the serving and preparation of meals. Nurses do their best to whet the appetite of those who have no inclination to eat, but on the whole they expect the patient's co-operation, if not gratitude for supplying him with food.

This is by no means the case in the psychiatric hospital, where a variety of feeding problems occur. There are patients who do not eat, or do not eat enough, or not the right kinds of food. Some patients eat too much, or too fast. Some eat each other's food, or bolt food without chewing it. There are those who no longer attach any social value to food, whose table manners are objectionable, or who perform rituals in such a way that food no longer serves as a social stimulus.

FOOD AND THE NURSE

The nurse can do a great deal in the treatment of her patients by giving meals the important place they deserve. Patients should be aware of meal-times and punctuality is important. There should be ample time before meals for patients to prepare for them, to put their things away, wash their hands and tidy up. Interest can be aroused by talking about food, discussing menus, exchanging recipes. Where possible, or desirable, patients may assist in the cooking of meals and, at any rate, in the laying of the tables. The meal itself should be a pleasurable occasion. It must be unhurried, nobody should disturb the harmony. Patients who may provide a disturbing influence may have to be served before or after the others, or in a separate dining-room. Patients who like each other should be placed next to each other and table conversation should be kept at a steady, leisurely flow. Meals should not produce anxiety, arguments should be avoided and any difficult situation which may arise over the feeding of resistive patients should be dealt with apart from others. The atmosphere of the dining-room should be congenial. The aesthetic pleasure of well-laid tables, well-cooked, well-served food cannot be ignored.

The nurse should think carefully about her own role in connection with meals. She should be the hostess who offers the food, not merely the 'maid' who carries it around. Meals must be served, but constant running in and fetching and carrying can have a very unsettling effect on patients. A nurse who remains in the dining-room, who can sit down with the patients at the table, can convey an attitude of relaxation and enjoyment, even if she is not sharing the meal.

The counting of cutlery is sometimes considered to be necessary but should not unduly disturb the atmosphere of the meal. By laying tables properly, so that each patient is given the same amount of cutlery, its checking is facilitated and it should not be impossible to keep after-dinner conversation going for a few moments while the cutlery is being counted.

It may be of some importance to decide whether meals should be served in the wards, or away from them in a central dining-room. The latter method usually has the advantage of providing hotter food, reducing delay between cooking and serving, and also of cutting down waste. Some patients enjoy the restaurant atmosphere of the dining-room, and benefit from a temporary absence from the ward. For other patients the ward for the time being represents 'home', the place to which he returns from work. Meals served in wards serve to draw patients closer to each other and thus to create the group feeling which should exist between patients and staff of the same ward.

In some hospitals attempts have been made to relieve nurses of purely domestic duties and it has been suggested that the work connected with the preparation for meals and the serving of food might be regarded as non-nursing and be delegated to the catering staff. While it may be a good idea to convey to some patients at certain times that they are independent of the nursing staff, that they are free to partake of restaurant meals as they see fit, that they can choose their menu and are free to miss a meal if they want to do so, it would seem quite wrong to believe that all meals should be regarded in this light. The act of serving food and accepting food has such powerful emotional significance that it provides a special opportunity for establishing important relationships between nurse and patient. When the patient is ready for greater independence it would seem advisable that he himself should assume greater responsibility for the provision of meals, rather than that other members of the staff should be drawn in. Facilities should exist for patients to prepare refreshments for entertainments, to entertain each other and their visitors, to go to the hospital canteen for a snack or to go out of the hospital and have tea in a restaurant in town.

Some patients can only gradually be brought into the community at meal-times, e.g. those who eat much more slowly than the rest, and have not finished in time, and those who may have to have their food cut up small, or minced; for example, epileptic patients who might have a fit while chewing large pieces of meat. Some patients may gobble their food, not giving themselves time to chew.

THE DIFFICULT PATIENT

By far the greatest skill, tact and perseverance is required when dealing with patients who refuse food. The method adopted to persuade these to eat must depend on the patient's motive for refusing food. Every effort should be made to discover individual problems in relation to food.

Many depressed patients are too apathetic to eat. There is no interest in food. The patient just does not want to be bothered, he is not hungry, has no desire for food. He would much rather be left alone and dislikes the nurse's attention. Sometimes, in order to rid himself of the nurse's attention, he may in fact attempt to eat but he is so slow that he may not receive an adequate diet. Only very careful observation will reveal the fact that such a patient has eaten or drunk far too little during the day. Regular weighing, careful attention to physical health, observation of bowel function, attention to the mouth, which may be dry due to lack of fluid intake, and sometimes the drawing up of intake and output charts, will provide an indication of the patient's state of nutrition. He may be merely passive, apathetic, uninterested, but he may not resist spoon-feeding, and it may be relatively easy to ensure adequate food and fluid intake.

Some patients, however, are quite determined not to eat. Some wish to commit suicide and believe starvation to be a suitable method. It is not too difficult to deal with this situation by kindly but firmly convincing the patient that this method cannot be allowed to succeed. Tube-feeding may be necessary once or twice to convince him, but often the nurse's own conviction that he will eat eventually is conveyed to him by word and bearing and makes him realize the futility of continuing to try to starve himself, although it may lead him to plan some alternative method of committing suicide.

Some depressed patients suffer from delusions which cause them to refuse food. The patient may have delusions of poverty or of unworthiness. He may believe that he does not have the money for his food, that he cannot eat what he cannot pay for, or else that he does not deserve it, is wicked, that other people are starving and food should be given to them. These ideas, expressed or kept secret by the patient, effectively deter him from eating. It will not help at all to tempt this patient with better or more expensive foods. Other methods must be employed. Sometimes it is possible, although perhaps not quite ethical, to accompany the patient in his delusion, and to suggest that it would be even more wicked to waste food, or to suggest that the nurse may find herself in trouble if the patient refuses food. The patient requires persuasion at every meal-time, and each time new and convincing reasons may have to be thought up as to why he should eat in spite of his alleged guilt or poverty.

The delusion that the patient has 'no inside', that his 'bowels are blocked' or that 'food turns to poison' inside him may lead to refusal of food. It is difficult to persuade the patient to eat and, having eaten, he is likely to vomit in order to avert the terrible consequences he feels would result from having food inside him. It may be necessary to be constantly with the patient after meals in order to prevent vomiting.

A patient may fear that he is being poisoned and consequently may refuse food from some members of the staff and accept it from others. He may consent to eat if he sees the food prepared or may eat if the nurse tastes the food first. He may insist on liquid or semi-solid food, which can be properly mixed before the nurse tastes the food. This may be repeated at every meal. Some patients may not reveal the reasons for refusal of food until they have recovered, and their unpredictable and erratic behaviour may puzzle nurses for a long time. Later the patient may explain that at times he had olfactory hallucinations which rendered the food suspect, or that he heard a voice telling him not to eat. He may have refused when offered with the right hand, but accepted it handed with the left, interpreting this as a sign that he should eat. Many bizarre delusions have a direct bearing on food intake.

Manic patients often refuse food because they are too busy and preoccupied with other things to be bothered with it. It may be possible to persuade such a patient to eat by putting food in his hand. He may for example eat a sandwich rather than a plateful of meat and vegetables.

It may be necessary to leave food about in the hope that it will be picked up and eaten.

Feeding difficulties of neurotic patients are particularly difficult to solve. In a similar manner to the child. the neurotic patient's refusal of food, or excessive food intake, may be an expression of his worry, anxiety and unhappiness.

As the patient's difficulties are resolved, so his appetite improves or becomes more normal. Meanwhile, however, the patient's physical health may suffer. It may be necessary to assist the process of recovery by using modified insulin therapy or continuous narcosis therapy to improve his condition, and thus to break the vicious circle of lack of nourishment, tiredness, listlessness, anorexia, giving rise to further malnutrition.

Some neurotic patients use meal-times in the way children do, as a weapon against authority, or as a means to attract attention. It is essential not only to find out what the patient is trying to achieve, but also why it is necessary for him to defy authority, or to attract notice in this way. Once it has been made clear to the patient, not so much in words but in attitude, that his motives are understood, that his attitude to authority is respected and his need for attention appreciated, he may be able to give up his symptom.

The patient's refusal of food may represent his attitude not to the nurse but to some other person whom she temporarily represents. His refusal of food may be a symbolic way of rejecting love, or rejecting care from a female who stands for a mother figure. It may indicate a fear of putting on weight which may be symbolic of a fear of pregnancy. It may be an expression of rebellion against dependence. Often a patient who refuses food can create differences of opinion among nurses, a situation which he can exploit but yet makes him feel insecure and unhappy.

Nurses sometimes feel that they must know the reason

for the patient's feeding problems in order to overcome them. It is helpful to know something about his motives, but often this is not possible because such motives are unconscious. They may become clear only as they are resolved. At best the nurse can make a guess and then act on the assumption that the guess is right. If she succeeds, she will think that the explanation was the right one. If she fails, the guess is rejected and she must try again. The guesses will become more nearly correct as the nurse tries varying approaches, listing those which succeed and those which fail. What is required of a nurse is not that she should know the reason of the patient's behaviour and act accordingly, but that she should be willing to try and find out. This willingness to understand in itself may convince the patient that the nurse is on his side and all problems may vanish.

The nurse who has failed to persuade the patient to eat should not regard this as a personal insult or feel that her failure will be regarded as incompetence. She must of course guard against interpreting another nurse's failure in this way. She must learn to observe other people's methods, compare them with her own and try to find out why one method or one person has failed and another succeeded. Sometimes she will continue to be puzzled until the patient himself, after recovery, can give her the real explanation.

CHAPTER 9

Socialization

It has already been shown that ward atmosphere plays an important part in the therapy of the patient and that it aims at creating an environment which is just right for the patients in that ward. When the patient has recovered, like any normal healthy person, he is able to manage difficulties, to live harmoniously with other people, to tolerate their weaknesses, to help and encourage those in need of help and to show sympathy and understanding for those in a more unfortunate position than himself.

During his stay he gains valuable experience in practising social skills by meeting in the same ward those who are suffering from mental illness of a different nature, those of different temperament and those who are less well than he is himself.

Patients' relatives often believe that it is bad for the patient to see others more seriously or more chronically ill than he is. They advocate some system of segregation of mentally ill patients into acute and chronic, or into mild and severe cases, but are reluctant to admit that their own relative belongs to the chronic or the severe group. They would wish to spare the mildly disturbed patient the sight of the more severely ill, yet agree that it is beneficial for the severeley disturbed patient to see others improving.

Many patients after treatment in a psychiatric hospital feel less prejudiced, ignorant and intolerant about the subject of mental illness than before treatment and probably much less so than their relatives and friends, who are so anxious to protect them from contact with other mentally ill patients.

There is no evidence that patients are harmed by being nursed in the same ward as others who are mentally ill. The right kind of atmosphere can be achieved even though the patients may vary greatly in many respects.

If all patients were severely disturbed it would be difficult to maintain a calm and normal atmosphere. The presence in the ward of some patients who are recovering provides the necessary stability and raises the morale of the ward.

Patients who are improving may derive a sense of security from witnessing how difficult situations are managed by the nurses. They may observe that a considerable degree of disturbed behaviour can be adequately contained, without disruption of the ward environment. Nurses remain calm and friendly despite provocation and continue to be genuinely interested in the disturbed patient although he may have insulted or attacked them. This may help the convalescent patient to realize that his own previously disturbed behaviour is not held against him.

Perhaps the only patients who suffer from contact with each other are manic patients. These are so easily stimulated that a ward containing more than one manic patient at any time is in constant danger of disruption. During an acute manic phase, in order to give the patient a maximal amount of rest and prevent exhaustion, it may be necessary to nurse him in a separate room or at least in a very quiet ward. Exposure to other equally noisy, restless patients could be harmful.

Other patients benefit by entering into social relationships with each other in the ward and valuable observational data can be obtained for diagnostic or therapeutic use.

Social Relationships Among Patients

Happiness is very largely linked with the ability to establish satisfying social relationships. Some people find it easy to make friends; others, as a result of rebuffs and failures, may have given up trying to do so. Rather than risk being rejected they make no attempt to be friendly. They do not know how to approach others, are so self-conscious and so worried about public opinion that they appear haughty, 'stuck up' and unapproachable and reject the very people whose friendship they would value. In normal life it is not always easy to make friends. Efforts must be made to meet people, go to parties, dances or clubs in order to make new acquaintances. But a person who has met with repeated failure, and who has found the attempt to make social contacts difficult and unrewarding, finds it simpler to remain at home and thereby becomes more and more solitary.

In hospital there is a very different situation. The patient inevitably finds himself in close association with others. He cannot escape contact with them and he has a unique opportunity of establishing some kind of social approach. He sleeps in the same room as other patients; bathes, washes and shaves, works side by side with them and shares the meal table with them. He has the same experiences, is subject to the same discipline, the same rules and routine. The same nurses and doctors care for many patients, the same entertainments are attended. The patient finds he has more interests in common with others than ever before, and it is therefore much easier to establish contact than it is in the outside world.

Furthermore, there is a variety of people available, some older and some younger, some more dependent than the patient and some more independent, some who can lead and some who wish to be led. The patient can experiment and often changes his friendships as he improves in health and is able to take responsibilities.

The patient is greatly helped in gaining confidence by the fact that he finds himself accepted in spite of his imagined or real shortcomings and in spite of his illness. Even if other patients at first reject him, the staff accept him whole-heartedly and befriend him. Sooner or later, he finds that he is accepted also by other patients. Generally speaking, knowledge of each other's illness and previous life brings patients closer together rather than causing them to reject each other. At first, tentatively, the patient confides in somebody expecting to be ridiculed and despised. If, instead, he finds that an interest is taken in him as a person, he gradually learns to trust others and to respect, in his turn, any confidence reposed in him. The patient's progress may be very slow and he may meet with many setbacks as the social structure of the ward changes.

THE NURSE'S ROLE

Nurses may fulfil the role of 'shock absorbers'. They form the stable, permanent element of the ward and hospital community; they can protect the patient from failure and prevent discouragement. For this purpose they should be aware of the patients' changing relationships in the group. It is important to know if any patient has friends and who these are. Friendships may arise between one patient who is dependent and seeks help and another who gives protection and support. This kind of friendship lasts only while each patient's needs are satisfied by it. As the more dependent patient improves and the other finds new outlets for his own potentialities, the association is dissolved. Changes in friendship, a knowledge of what has caused the separation, an awareness of the needs which are satisfied by ward friendships can provide useful indications of progress.

The Patient and the Group

The patient's relationship to the group as a whole is important. He may feel that he 'belongs' and is accepted by others, and may derive benefit from his popularity. Whether he emerges as leader or assumes a subordinate role may depend on his personality and may indicate the kind of social setting most congenial to him.

If he remains an outsider and is not accepted by the group, he may, feeling himself hostile and rejected, require the help of the nurse to restore his self-confidence, raise his opinion of himself and at the same time become aware of his own attitudes to group membership. When he is ready to join he may require the help and support of a nurse to make the first move.

When difficult situations arise in the ward the patient's attitude to the staff may give an indication of his progress. Jealousies between patients who have the same doctor, or competition for the attention of the ward sister, may indicate the patient's dependence on the hospital. His growing sense of security may manifest itself in the manner in which he identifies himself with the group of patients. As a member of the ward group he may for the first time find courage to criticize the hospital or those in authority. He may become less frightened of his feeling of rebellion, able to understand his attitude and to revise it. Gradually his growing social awareness may lead to a sense of belonging to the ward as a whole. Co-operation with others may replace dependence or self-assertion. The patient may understand the emotional interaction which takes place between staff, other patients and himself and he may be able to use his newly won confidence in order to help other patients who are less well.

Gradually the patient ventures beyond the immediate circle of the ward. In the occupation departments and at entertainments he meets patients from other wards and he has wider scope for the practice of social skills. Eventually he looks for friends outside the hospital.

It helps greatly if opportunity is provided for patients to take an active part in making decisions in the ward and in the hospital as a whole. Regular meetings of patients in the ward provide the opportunity to state opinions and express feelings. Patients gain courage, confidence and prestige by being able to speak in public and finding that others listen with interest. If some meetings are conducted in a fairly formal manner patients can practise taking the office of chairman or secretary and benefit from having to take responsibility.

Hospital entertainments, sports events and other inter ward activities can usefully be organized by patients' committees. To be elected by the other patients in the ward to be a representative and spokesman can be a very gratifying experience and many patients are surprised at their own competence once the opportunity for using initiative is provided.

The hospital can help in the transition by providing ex-patient and out-patient clubs, thus giving such support as the individual patient needs until he is convinced of his own unaided ability to establish social relationships.

CHAPTER 10

Occupation—A Therapeutic Tool

To a large extent the patient's progress can be judged by his eagerness and ability to work. Work is an essential therapeutic tool in psychiatry. This fact has long been recognized by psychiatrists and nurses alike and in all psychiatric hospitals provision is now made for a large variety of occupations, designed to suit different people at various stages of their illness. Although many hospitals employ occupational therapists and craftsmen to instruct patients and supervise work in the workshops and occupational therapy departments, it is nearly always the nurse's task to ensure the success of the arrangements in operation at the hospital.

Two functions in particular should be carried out by the nurse; first, to ensure that the patient has both knowledge and conviction that the occupation is truly therapeutic and, second, to provide him with sufficient incentive to undertake work. Her ingenuity added to any special talent she may possess are often invaluable in stimulating interest. The nurse co-operates with psychiatrist and occupational therapists in making sure that the right kind of occupation is found for each patient.

WORK AND SOCIETY

It is well to remember the importance of work in normal life. For most people it occupies the greater part of every day. The vast majority have to work to a regular time-table, arriving in the morning at the correct time and carrying out a full day's work. Most people have to mix with others during their working day. They work side by side with colleagues, co-operate with them on a single job, or compete with them in doing what has to be done. They may have to take orders from superiors, submit to criticism, sometimes unjustified, and accept correction. They may have to give orders to others, and criticize or correct the work of those in subordinate positions.

People do all these things in order to earn their living, to take responsibility for their families and to enable them to devote the rest of their time to the enjoyment of their leisure in pursuits such as sports, games, theatres, music and travelling. Many people require special incentives in their work; wages, shorter hours, better working conditions. Many others, however, derive pleasure from work itself. They have chosen their occupations in such a way that work provides them with full satisfaction and few extraneous incentives are needed. Others, again, care little for money incentives, they work best when they know that their efforts are useful and appreciated by others. Whatever the main incentive, the working man is making a very difficult and complex adjustment, not only to the work situation as such, but to his family who benefit by his work, and to society which expects him to work in return for the benefits it bestows upon him.

WORK IN MENTAL ILLNESS

For one reason or another, a patient who is mentally ill may find it no longer possible to cope with work. An individual may fail in many ways in adaptation, but society takes the most serious view of the person who is incapable of working.

Very frequently the history of a patient reveals an unsatisfactory adjustment to work. Some patients have a very poor work record, frequent changes of jobs having been made, always for trifling reasons. Some have gradually deteriorated in efficiency and attendance over a period of time. Some have broken down when faced with new responsibilities, others have held jobs too simple and monotonous for their intelligence. Some housewives have neglected their family and simply stayed in bed, refusing to do anything at all. People who behave like this suffer financial loss, lose the esteem of their family and friends and their prestige vanishes. They are criticized, exhorted and advised, they are made to feel the consequences of their behaviour.

When the patient comes into hospital, he is accepted as being ill, not wicked or lazy. Whether he works or not, he is looked after, cared for and receives attention. He lacks nothing. The nurse tries to convince him that he is liked and esteemed whether he works or not. With the help of the social worker his family is given support. Material incentives are removed.

Although there is no need to work in order to earn a living, the patient is expected to work as part of his treatment. The only reward offered is the intrinsic value of the work itself, the increasing self-esteem and the pleasure his family derives from seeing him recover.

Work as an Aid to Treatment

It is essential that the work should be most carefully planned by all those who are trying to help the patient and by the patient himself. Every success on the patient's part must be acknowledged. He must be offered every opportunity to increase his scope. Realistic, lifelike work situations of increasing difficulty are provided and he is encouraged to tackle them. Yet, if he fails, he is protected from the consequences of failure. He is encouraged to look forward to taking up proper employment and should never be allowed to feel that it would be better to give up trying. Even for the patient who remains in hospital, full employment to the best of his ability should be the aim, because without satisfying full-time work the patient gets bored and loses his sense of independence.

The first consideration when finding suitable work for a patient is the usefulness of what he is doing. Some patients produce articles for themselves or as presents for their family. This provides a means of retaining contact and a certain degree of responsibility. The nurse should always know for whom the article is designed, and should encourage the patient's endeavours by referring to the pleasure it will give his wife or child to receive the gift. It may be necessary to discuss with the wife how helpful it is for the patient that she should register pleasure when she receives it. If the patient is despondent and feels rejected by his family, the nurse may encourage him to work for her. He may sweep or dust to please the nurse, do odd jobs, or make a cushion if he knows one is needed in his ward. As the patient improves, he may be encouraged to work for the hospital or for others who are not as well as he is. His work should be appreciated and at every step he should be aware of its usefulness.

The patient should be successful in his work. His previous occupation, abilities and ambitions are taken into consideration and work which he can do is provided. Sometimes it would be unwise to allow him to work in line with his usual employment because he might then set himself standards which are too high. However well he does the work while he is ill, it is likely to compare unfavourably with his real work at its best. This comparison would serve only to confirm in his mind the fact that he is a failure.

Normally people set a certain aim and hope to achieve something which is just a little bit difficult. Success leads to rejoicing and the level of aspiration is raised a little higher. Sometimes failure acts as a spur to greater effort. Mentally ill patients sometimes have quite unrealistic aims. Many set themselves such high standards that they are bound to suffer failure. Others are so despondent that they do not try anything which is not well below their known standard of ability. In encouraging the patient to work, he needs help to adjust his standards. The nurse can help him with troublesome details in order to ensure success. Only very gradually should the patient be made responsible for dealing with his own mistakes and encouraged to tackle difficulties. Work should be found for him which he can finish by himself. If the task takes too long he will become discouraged and perhaps cease trying. The nurse should be entirely clear as to whether to expect perfection from a particular patient or whether to accept inferior workmanship for the sake of seeing an endeavour brought to its proper conclusion.

The Time Factor in Work

For certain patients the hours of working may be an important factor to be considered rather than the work itself. Some who are obsessional may find it almost impossible to arrive anywhere in time and may have to concentrate on time rather than on the work to be done in the occupational therapy department. To psychopaths regular attendance may provide the main problem, while schizophrenic or hypomanic patients may find it difficult to concentrate for long on one job. The occupation time should be planned for each patient individually. Some patients are responsible for arriving at work unaccompanied and doing so regularly and punctually. Others are accompanied to the occupation department. The number of hours of work varies according to the patient's age and the degree of his illness. In each case it must be decided whether to overlook frequent interruptions and rest pauses, or whether it is important that the patient should be kept busy all the time.

GROUP WORKING

Work may contribute considerably towards the socialization of the patient. He may work alone, alongside others or on a project with other patients, he may have to take instructions from others or be made responsible for the work of a group. The domestic work in the ward, for instance, can be so arranged that each patient does his job with a minimum of communication with others, or it may be. arranged in such a way that real team spirit prevails. Under such conditions, the patients interact with each other and a leader usually emerges or may be appointed. Valuable observations can be 'made about the patients' relationships to one another and each has an opportunity, in the shelter of a hospital environment, to try out techniques of interpersonal relationships.

The kinds of occupations provided depend on the arrangements made available at the hospital. Existing facilities should be used to the best advantage of individual patients. Domestic work in the ward or in other departments, kitchen work, carpentry, upholstery, brushmaking, shoemaking, sewing, tailoring, are available in most hospitals. Gardens, farms, arts and crafts departments, laundry and bakery offer suitable work to some patients.

It is usually most difficult to find suitable employment for patients who dislike or resent manual work. These may be encouraged to help with typing or in the library. They may help with educational classes for other patients. Sometimes, however, patients from professional fields of work settle down remarkably well to almost any job they are asked to do, provided they can see its usefulness or creativity.

Occupational retraining may be necessary after prolonged stay in a psychiatric hospital or if the patient's illness has left him partially disabled. Various industrial retraining schemes which have been introduced in psychiatric hospitals are discussed in Chapter 14.

PAYMENT FOR WORK

If the patient has been in hospital for a long time it may be advisable to offer payment for work. The idea of working competitively may be associated with financial reward. Where piece work is carried out the patient can measure his own improvement and money acts as incentive for better output. More important still, some patients may have forgotten the value of money. Budgeting, planning how to spend, learning how much things cost, may be an important aspect of rehabilitation.

Except in these circumstances it is doubtful whether monetary reward should ever be used as an incentive for work. Patients may rightly feel that they are being used as cheap labour if they are capable of doing a job well but receive only pocket money. If they are not able to work well, the training, supervision, encouragement and assistance they receive is all part of their treatment and it is therefore quite inappropriate for them to be paid. If the nurse is involved in evaluating the patient's work for purposes of payment, and even more so if she is actively required to pay the patient, it becomes impossible for her to maintain a therapeutic relationship with him.

CHAPTER 11

Rest, Exercise, Recreation, Sleep

———

THE patient spends a considerable period of his time at work in one or other of the occupational therapy departments of the hospital. Some of his time, varying in amount according to his age and illness, is spent in attending to personal hygiene and to meals. The remaining time is given to exercise, recreational activities, rest and sleep.

SLEEP

It is essential for the patient's physical health that he should have adequate, deep, restful sleep.

Insomnia

Many patients complain that for a long time prior to admission they have suffered from 'insomnia'. Careful inquiries show that there are many ways in which sleep can be disturbed. Some patients say that they have not slept a wink for many weeks. This is unlikely to be true, but the complaint should be listened to by the nurse, because it is an indication of the patient's suffering and distress. He may attribute his many symptoms to lack of sleep. He is worried, anxious and frightened. This keeps him awake at night. But he believes that he is worried, anxious and frightened *because* he cannot sleep, and expresses fear of going 'mad' if he does not soon find relief. It is useless to point out to him that there is evidence of his having slept for certain periods; it is much better to listen to his complaint and ask him for details of his insomnia.

Insomnia is very widespread in the community as a whole. General Practitioners prescribe a very large amount of sedation.

Studies of sleep patterns have shown that the amount of sleep people enjoy diminishes with age; complaints of insomnia increase with age.

The satisfaction derived from sleep depends on the length of sleep and on the depth of sleep. The electro-encephalograph shows a variety of brain waves during sleep. The wave pattern in deep sleep is slow. Although only short periods of the night may be spent in sleep with slow-wave pattern, the satisfaction reported in the morning is associated with this type of sleep. When the brainwaves are shallow and fast, there is a subsequent feeling of not having slept well. Efficiency during the day appears to depend to some extent on the amount of sleep during which slow brainwaves occurred.

During part of the sleeping period the sleeper's eyes move rapidly and the E.E.G. record shows rapid eye movement. Waking the sleeper at this moment makes it clear that he has been disturbed in the middle of a dream. If people are deprived of the opportunity of dreaming, they also complain of a poor night's sleep.

The patient's own account and complaints may therefore be justified, even when the night nurse's observation indicates that the patient slept for longer periods than he is aware of.

Some patients fall asleep quite easily in the evening, but wake frequently and remain awake for long periods. To the patient, the wakeful periods seem endless, the periods of sleep pass unnoticed or by comparison appear to be short.

Patients who are anxious and frightened find it difficult to go to sleep in the evening. Once asleep, they sleep soundly and do not wake again until morning. But the early hours of the night are agony. The more the patient tries to sleep, the more anxious, and therefore the more wakeful, he becomes. Rather than suffer these dreadful hours, the patient prefers to remain up and dressed, and like a child practises delaying tactics in the evening. He may take a long time undressing, go back again and again for something he has forgotten, fold clothes meticulously and repeatedly, fetch water and hot-water bottles and generally make bedtime difficult for all. If he is harassed and nagged, his anxiety increases and his sleeplessness becomes worse. It is better to convince him that his difficulties are appreciated and that the nurse will be near and will help him fall asleep.

Some patients, especially those who are depressed, wake up very early in the morning and at that time find life quite intolerable. The early hours of the morning might then become the most propitious time for an attempt at suicide.

Nightmares

Many mentally ill patients suffer from nightmares. The patient may wake during the night terrified, in a cold sweat and trembling. He requires someone to be near in order to bring him back gently to reality and to tell him that he had a nightmare, a bad dream, and that he is quite safe. The patient may wish to speak about his dream, or he may just want a nurse to sit by him for a few moments until he has calmed down. Dreams play an important part in the manifestations and treatment of mentally ill patients. It may be very desirable for the patient to remember his dreams and to tell either his doctor or the nurse, who could write it down for him.

Naturally, after a bad night, the patient feels tired all day. He seeks every opportunity to lie down on his bed, lacks energy and inclination for work. He may doze off to sleep, so getting some badly needed rest, but finding it all the more difficult to sleep the following night.

Factors influencing Sleep

Many sleep disturbances are symptomatic of psychiatric disorders. Often, however, the patient's inability to sleep is caused by conditions in the hospital ward. Most people find it disturbing to sleep in a room with others, especially strangers. Some dormitories in psychiatric hospitals are so crowded, beds are so close to each other, that it is not surprising that patients sleep badly. Patients who in their own home have interior-sprung mattresses or latex-foam beds may be expected to sleep on hard hospital beds, often with a mackintosh under the sheet. Pillows may be hard or arranged in an unaccustomed manner, blankets too few or too many. Patients who are used to open windows find the ward stuffy, others complain of draught.

Most patients, at least during the first few nights, complain of noise; they are aware of the breathing and snoring of others, of the footsteps of the nurse, the whispered talk in the corridors, the ringing of telephone bells and the clanking noise of crockery in the kitchen. The light is left on during the night, disturbing to some patients although it is subdued, and disturbing to others who would prefer bright lights because they are frightened by shadows and the dim outlines of furniture.

It is the first and foremost duty of the night nurse to minimize disturbing factors in the ward and to realize that these are not the same for all patients.

It is impossible to over-emphasize the importance of silence in the ward, of ventilation and warmth, of comfortable, well-made beds, remade if the patient is restless. Needless to say, the patient should not be allowed to go hungry or lack water to drink. Hot drinks may help and he may find relief if he gets up to empty bowels or bladder, or merely to change his position.

To the patient it is not only important that all things should be done to ensure a quiet night, it is important *how* they are done. The way in which the nurse offers him a drink, or remakes his bed, is often more important than the actual drink or bedmaking. The presence of the night nurse may be all that is required in order to re-assure the patient. If the nurse is not in evidence, he calls out so as to reassure himself of her presence and, having called, he is bound to ask for something. The nurse should understand this need, and be present even if the patient does not require any attention. She should inform patients of her movements, tell them that she will be in the ward, explain how they can attract her attention. If she goes away from the ward to her meal, she should tell the patients about this, and also mention who will be there to relieve her.

In order to ensure that patients obtain a good night's sleep, the routine of the ward must be so arranged that all have adequate amounts of exercise and fresh air during the day. The retiring hour should be suited to each ward and ample time should be allowed for gradual preparation for bed. There should be a reduction in noise and excitement before bedtime and a period of quiet relaxation.

Flexible arrangements for retiring are very helpful. Some people habitually retire late and read for a while before switching off the lights. They find this helps to get to sleep quickly.

It is not always essential that a patient who is wakeful should remain in bed. To sit in the dayroom reading, or to talk to the night nurse for a while may be more helpful than efforts to go to sleep.

It is incumbent on the day staff to read the night report, and to increase exercise and activity during the day if it seems indicated by poor sleep at night.

Spectacles should not be taken away from patients. There is nothing more irritating to a patient with poor eyesight than to be without his glasses, unable to read, unable to watch what is going on, and unable to sleep because of the general noise and activity.

Sedation

If, in spite of all these nursing measures, the patient does not sleep, or complains of not sleeping, the nurse should keep a careful record. Every half-hour she should check whether the patient is awake or asleep, and in the report she should not only state the number of hours of sleep, but give an account of sleep rhythm and quality. Sedatives are quite freely used in the treatment of mental disorder, but the right sedative can be prescribed only if the doctor is fully informed of the patient's sleeping habits and of the effect of the drug. The nurse should know if the sedative prescribed for the patient is quick or slow acting and whether or not it has prolonged effects. This is particularly important with drugs to be given 's.o.s.', or to be repeated. She should know how late it is desirable to give any drug, and how long she can delay, in order to give the patient a chance to sleep without sedation.

REST, EXERCISE AND RECREATION

Rest

Well-meaning friends and relatives often try to help in the early stages of psychiatric illness by advising a rest, a change or a holiday. The patient rarely benefits, and if, after an expensive holiday, he feels as weak and ill as before, he becomes more discouraged and more trying to his family.

Provided the patient has a good night's sleep, rest during the day is rarely indicated in psychiatric illness, unless the patient's physical condition demands it. Old people like to rest for a short time after luncheon and of course require frequent short rest pauses after any physical exertion, such as climbing stairs or helping with ward cleaning.

Any patient who is losing weight should, in addition to other remedial measures, have periods of rest in bed. Very often this is achieved by putting the patient on modified insulin treatment or on continuous narcosis. It is rarely desirable to allow or encourage patients to sit about or lie on beds, unoccupied, listless and idle.

Normal healthy people are usually fully occupied during their leisure time. It is a common complaint of healthy people that leisure is all too short for their many hobbies and interests. It is a sign of ill health to be incapable of enjoying leisure, to be disinclined to do anything at all, wishing to remain idle and unoccupied and feeling a need for rest. The extent to which a mentally ill patient is occupied and the way in which he plans his leisure is one of the surest indications of progress during his stay in hospital.

People's tastes and interests vary considerably and it would take many pages to list all the activities which people find interesting enough to occupy them in their spare time. In hospital something for all tastes should be provided. While the patient's likes and dislikes for a particular form of occupation should be respected, all patients should be encouraged to try everything once. Many patients acquire new and absorbing interests during their hospital stay which help them later when, after discharge, they again encounter difficult situations.

The amount of leisure time available varies from ward to ward. Where patients are fully occupied with occupational therapy only evenings are free, apart from brief periods after meals. Where patients take longer over meals, washing, dressing and toilet, there is less free time than there is in wards where patients are young and energetic. A time-table of free periods should be drawn up and the best possible use made of these.

Exercise

It is essential that every patient should spend a part of each day out of doors. If the weather is very good, occupational therapy sessions are often held in the open air. The colder the weather, the more thought and planning is necessary, because then the patients have to change their shoes, and put on overcoats, gloves and hats before going for walks. All this can be very time-consuming, and unless organization is good, much time is wasted looking for patients, opening doors, dressing and undressing. If patients go out as a group, the time for the walk should be generally known to everyone well in advance. By repeatedly mentioning the fact that a walk is planned, and reminding patients of the hour of departure, the nurse can reduce the time spent in persuading patients to go, and in preparing for it. It is important to be as quick as possible once the first patient is ready. There should be no hanging around and waiting for each other. It is annoying for the patient, who has reluctantly dressed himself to go out, to be kept waiting for a quarter of an hour or more for others.

If the weather is cold, it is important to ensure that no patient becomes chilled as a result of standing about or sitting down outside in very cold weather.

If the weather is good, garden doors are often kept open. The nurse should know which patients are outside. For a short time, patients are content to sit and enjoy the sunshine, or to walk about without specific aim. After that boredom sets in, and the patients may just stand or sit in a withdrawn, lethargic manner, as they might do indoors. Out of doors there are added physical risks to be guarded against, such as sunburn, insect stings or bites, and possible damage to the eyes from dust or bright sunlight.

Some outdoor activities should be part of the ward routine. Instead of walking round and round, outdoor games should be arranged. Tennis, rounders or other ball games may be played. Some patients find enjoyment in watching. Running or jumping may be practised. Inter-ward cricket and football matches and inter-ward athletics are usually popular, both for those who participate and for those who watch and take sides. Some patients play games for the first time since their schooldays and they are often surprised how well they are still able to do this and how much they enjoy the game. Participation in team games is of importance for reasons quite apart from the opportunity afforded of enjoying fresh air.

In some hospitals, country walks or shopping walks are arranged. Not every patient is able to join in, but, for those able to undertake them, walks outside the hospital boundary form a link with the outside world and a stepping-stone towards discharge. Usually it is the nurse's responsibility to decide who should be taken for a walk, and the success of the venture depends upon the accuracy of her selection. It is usually safe to take a group of about twenty patients with two nurses, provided none of the patients is suicidal or likely to run away, but smaller groups are desirable if the occasion is to be enjoyed to the full. If any suicidal patients are in the party an extra nurse may be required. The walk should be planned in the same way as a guide taking a party of tourists plans the walk. Having assessed the patients' physical stamina, the route is planned. If possible, it is timed, and the distance is not beyond the powers of any patient. The patients should know where they are going and, if possible, some preliminary discussion should take place, so that as each landmark is reached a feeling of being familiar with the countryside is engendered. There should be a definite aim, a particular place to be reached, chosen for its beauty, its suitability for a picnic or for its historical interest. If there is no particular goal some patients begin to agitate and want to return before the others and the general morale falls. This does not happen if all know where they are going and if, on arrival, there is a short rest, perhaps a cup of tea and then the return journey.

Many interests can be fostered during country walks, and any special knowledge of particular patients should be used to the fullest extent. If a patient is an expert botanist he should be encouraged to tell others about the flowers of the district, to point out rare flowers, perhaps help to collect some, and perhaps give another talk on return. Historians can encourage interest in historical places, patients with a knowledge of architecture may interest others in the style of buildings in the district, and bird-watchers may communicate to fellow patients their own pleasure in observing birds.

The nurses who are with the group should arrange with each other what each should do. They should leave word at the hospital where they have taken the patients and when they intend to return. One should lead the party and the second keep well to the back. In traffic it may be wise to walk on the kerbside of the pavement, near water on the water side of the path. Bridges, road crossings, traffic, all represent special danger points. The nurse should notice if a patient frequently stoops to pick up something and she should investigate and prevent the hoarding of rubbish or the collection of poisonous plants or berries.

Arrangements should be made in advance as to which nurse should remain behind in the case of an accident, and which one should continue on her way with the patients. If this is not done, panic and arguments may arise if, for instance, a patient slips and injures his ankle, and while the nurses are deciding who should remain to render first aid other patients may come to harm. After return, the walk remains for some time a topic of conversation, and nurses can use the enthusiasm of patients to interest others in future similar walks.

Leisure Time Activities

Apart from making sure that all patients spend some time of the day out of doors, leisure time should be so arranged that the patient's background, interests and ability are taken into account. Every effort should be made to encourage the taking up of new interests and hobbies and the trying out, while in hospital, of activities which may be useful after discharge. It is characteristic of many forms of mental ill-health that the patient is unable to plan or enjoy his leisure, and unable also to obtain from it the relaxation he needs. Sometimes the patient complains that overwork makes it impossible for him to devote any time to leisure activities and he explains his gradual social isolation to himself and others as being the result of his work. But in reality he drives himself to work, in order to avoid his social obligations. He deprives himself of free time, which would expose his inability profitably to occupy his leisure.

Many patients have experienced repeated failure in their attempts to establish social contacts and they have failed miserably to feel at ease in company. They desperately want to be liked, to make friends, to relax and feel happy with others. They envy those who are admired, popular and surrounded by friends. They may often have steeled themselves to attend dances or parties, always hoping to enjoy them, always pretending to have done so, but becoming increasingly discouraged, self-conscious and shy, until finally they feel quite unable ever again to make the effort and shudder at the very thought of attending social gatherings.

Social Activities

Hospital parties are well suited to help the patient to gain courage and to be successful where previously he has failed. It is, however, no easy matter to persuade such a patient to make the first attempt, and in no circumstances must a failure be risked. It is often advisable to run dancing classes and to take the patient to these, acting as partner, until he feels sufficiently self-confident to risk a dance. By then he may have met one or two of the other patients in a situation resembling a social occasion and may not feel entirely strange when he eventually attends a dance.

Hospital dances should be enjoyed by all who attend; all who like dancing should be given the opportunity to do so. There should be no 'wallflowers', and male and female nurses should ask those patients to dance who have not been approached by others or do not have the courage to ask a partner. Dances in hospital usually last a short time compared with those held outside and they rapidly get into swing. There should be a good Master of Ceremonies who makes use of introducing dances where all can join in. Square dancing or Paul Jones give an opportunity even for the shyest to take part. It may be advisable to arrange dances with predominantly 'Old-Time' dancing for older patients, and other dances with opportunity for contemporary dances for younger people. Dances should be well prepared in advance. The patients need adequate time to devote to their toilet. If possible, special party clothes should be available and every encouragement given to patients to make themselves as attractive as possible. After the dance, the patients will wish to discuss their experiences, and nurses can use the opportunity to emphasize success and to prepare the way for even greater success the next time.

While it is extremely important for the nurse to assist some patients to enjoy dancing, and so to gain courage to attend dances after their discharge, there will be many patients who have no wish to dance and who find other forms of entertainment more congenial. For this reason the greatest variety of entertainments should be available. Some patients relax best at informal socials. They may enjoy party games and may seek new ideas with which to entertain their friends, later gaining prestige and becoming active rather than passive members at a social occasion.

Not all entertainments should allow patients to remain passive. Socials should be organised by the patients in turn. Many patients derive satisfaction from arranging a party, acting as hosts to others, preparing refreshments. Patients may learn to co-operate with each other to make the party a success. Some have the opportunity of taking up leadership, emerging as efficient, capable organizers. Provided the nurses join in, most patients are able to contribute in some way towards the enjoyment of the occasion. Experience of working for a common goal provides a tie among the members of the ward, gives a feeling of unity and solidarity, and helps to raise the morale of the ward.

Radio parlour games can be imitated as ward entertainments. Such games as 'Twenty Questions' or 'What's My Line' give a number of patients an opportunity for active participation. At all these forms of entertainment the patients mix with those from other wards, make friends, develop social graces and at the same time acquire social skills which may be of considerable use after discharge. However, many patients are left unsatisfied by such forms of entertainment and there should be as many varied kinds of social activities and entertainments as possible in order to give all patients something of interest. No talent should be wasted and every nurse should make it her aim to find something for all of her patients. The slightest hint on the part of a nurse, a word of encouragement, or a creative idea, may encourage some patient to find a new purpose in life. The more unusual the patient's interest, the more he needs a nurse who shares and appreciates it.

Patients value a proper balance between 'going out' and 'staying at home'. Records, radio and television give much pleasure to some patients, but the choice of programme needs careful thought. The young, energetic members of the community need opportunities for developing their interest in 'pop' songs and rhythmic noise, without disturbing the older members or those whose tastes differ. Patients who appreciate serious music or who wish to listen to plays or follow educational programmes should have facilities for doing so.

Where space permits it may be helpful to reserve a room, or part of a room, for those who watch television, leaving the rest of the ward free for other activities, or alternatively to reserve one room for those who wish to have peace and quiet while noisy activities go on elsewhere. In some wards patients in their meetings can scrutinize the radio and television programmes for the week and arrive at some agreement about the times when the set shall be switched on. It is always helpful if nurses take an interest in radio, television and record programmes and join the patients in discussions before and after; for very often talking about the previous night's viewing can be the most valuable aspect of television. Often it is possible to develop interests which have been stimulated by television.

Among the activities which take place within the wards are games of cards, chess, draughts, jigsaw puzzles, solving of crossword puzzles or quizzes. These activities can be particularly valuable in helping to establish personal relationships between nurse and patient or between patients. They offer patients the opportunity of gradual approach to other people. A game of cards can just be watched, the patient tentatively approaching an existing group without too many demands being made on him. He can at first play a silent game with a nurse and very gradually allow himself to get close. Skilled nurses can gradually introduce other patients into the group and gradually withdraw when the patient is able to feel comfortable in a group of patients.

Parties organized by patients in the ward are often greatly enjoyed. Patients' birthdays can be celebrated in some special way, without necessarily having parties for all. It is quite important that the patient whose birthday is celebrated should feel that he is the centre of attention and the cause of the celebration. Birthday cards admired by all, specially chosen food for lunch, first choice in deciding what should be done in the evening, a birthday cake, can be of more value than elaborate parties.

Because patients who are mentally disturbed find it difficult to organize their own leisure, much thought should be given to the use of leisure by the nursing staff. However, arrangements should never be made for the patient, without involving him at every stage in planning and in making decisions. Many entertainments are enjoyed much more if one has time to think about them ahead. As soon as possible the patient should have an opportunity of planning, for himself, how he wishes to spend his spare time.

As patients recover, more unorganized time is needed for private and personal pursuits. Reading newspapers, writing letters, reading books, or quiet chats with other patients may become more important and more valuable than organized activities. There is in some hospitals a serious problem of shortage of space and patients may complain that it is difficult to find a quiet spot and privacy.

Provision of libraries or reading rooms in hospital may be of value, and sometimes patients can find peace in the ward while others are at work or away from the ward at organized entertainments.

Books for Further Reading

J. Burr. (1967) *Nursing the Psychiatric Patient*. Baillière, Tindall & Cassell, London.

G. K. Hoffling and M. M. Leininger. (1960) *Basic Psychiatric Concepts in Nursing*. Lippincott, Philadelphia.

M. Ingram. (1965) *Principles of Psychiatric Nursing*. Saunders, Philadelphia.

M. E. Kalkman. (1958) *Introduction to Psychiatric Nursing.* McGraw-Hill, New York.

D. C. Maddison, P. Day and B. Leadbeater. (1965) *Psychiatric Nursing.* 2nd ed. Livingstone, Edinburgh.

M. L. Manfreda. (1964) *Psychiatric Nursing.* F. A. Davis, Philadelphia.

R. Matheney and M. Topalis. (1965) *Psychiatric Nursing.* 4th ed. Kimpton, London.

CHAPTER 12

Nursing Disturbed Children
and Adolescents

———

SOME general principles underlying the care of psychiatrically disturbed patients have been described so far.

In this and the following chapters some of the principles will be discussed with reference to certain groups of patients, for whom special provisions are necessary.

Children and adolescents, for whom an increasing number of hospitals are setting aside wards for their treatment, are two such groups.

Although not all psychiatric nurses will have the opportunity of nursing children or adolescents, they may be interested to know something about the essential aspects of caring for these patients.

Disturbance in children can manifest itself first at home or at school. All children pass through difficult phases at some time or other and it may be extremely difficult to decide whether a child's behaviour necessitates professional help or not. For brief periods disturbed behaviour is usually tolerated, though considerable anxiety may be aroused. Parental anxiety may then in turn result in increased disturbance in the child's behaviour.

When the child's disturbance becomes severe or goes on for a long time parents may feel under increased pressure to seek guidance and help.

Help is available from a number of sources. There are child guidance clinics associated with education authorities, where an educational psychologist assesses the child's problems and either treats the child or obtains psychiatric advice.

When the general practitioner is first consulted by the parents the child may be referred to a psychiatrist in a paediatric or psychiatric out-patient department. In psychiatric clinics associated with the health services it is usual for a psychiatrist and psychologist to see the child for diagnosis and treatment. A psychiatric social worker helps the parents with their problems.

Children's officers and probation officers, who in the past only became concerned with disturbed children and adolescents after a breakdown in the home had occurred, are increasingly charged with prevention. Children and adolescents may be referred to them in the first instance, and they may be able to give the necessary support with or without consultation of a psychiatrist.

In-patient treatment in hospital is only rarely resorted to. Treatment as out-patients or in special day or boarding schools for maladjusted children is much more frequent. Even when a period of in-patient treatment is necessary this is only a short episode in a much longer phase of treatment outside. The health of the whole family must therefore always be considered when a child is referred for psychiatric treatment.

In the case of children, psychotherapy sometimes takes the form of indirect interviews. The child finds it difficult to explain his worries and fears but he can talk about them more freely while he s playing, painting or drawing. His use of toys in the playroom indicates the stage of his development, and the nature of his disturbance. Observing the child at play reveals whether he plays constructively or destructively, whether he is relaxed or tense, inhibited or imaginative, friendly or hostile. Playing with dolls may reveal his feelings about various people.

Some of the children seen in clinics are mentally

retarded. Often the anxiety of parents about the late development of a child causes emotional disturbances which are the real reason for seeking help. Reassurance and arrangements for special training and special treatment may enable the parents to accept the limitations of the child and when excessive demands are no longer made on him, he may again settle down.

THE DIFFICULTIES OF DIAGNOSIS

Among the children who show disturbed behaviour necessitating treatment are those who may be suffering from early psychotic illnesses, those whose difficulties are associated with brain damage, epilepsy, or encephalitic infections, and those whose disturbed behaviour is closely related to mistakes in upbringing, to emotional disturbances in the family and to materal unhappiness and anxiety. Many children come from broken homes, some are orphans, many have suffered separation from the mother during the first few years of life.

It is difficult to diagnose clearly any particular form of psychiatric illness in children. Many of the symptoms which are found in sick children are similar to those found in psychotic or neurotic adults, but some symptoms, which would be serious in adults, may be perfectly normal at least at some stage of childhood. Withdrawal into phantasy, giggling and posturing, which would indicate a schizophrenic illness in adults, are not abnormal in early adolescence. Compulsive rituals are common in small children and form part of many games played even by those who are older. Showing off is common, interest in the body, display and exposure are characteristic stages of development in most children, especially girls. No single symptom can be taken as evidence of mental disorder in a child. Even where the child's total behaviour pattern is definitely maladjusted it is difficult to decide if the illness is a reaction to a current emotional disturbance in the parents, evidence of the development of a neurotic personality, or an early psychotic manifestation.

Children are easily influenced by environmental changes. Much suffering among them is the result of reaction to tensions experienced in the home. Children also influence their environment and much parental unhappiness and tension is caused by the maladjustment of a child.

Symptoms in children are as much determined by their age and stage of development, as by the specific disorder from which the child suffers.

At every stage of development the child is capable of only a limited repertoire of behaviour and disturbance can occur only in such aspects of behaviour. In very young children the most common manifestations of disturbance affect sleep and feeding. Later, difficulties arise with elimination. All these are referred to as habit disorders.

As the child grows older it normally becomes interested in the physical environment. Play is important in the development of physical skills and intellectual progress. At this stage some children manifest their disturbance in apathy, lack of curiosity and failure to play; others play wildly and restlessly with such persistent overactivity that little progress is possible. Speech development is often disturbed and consequently the child's ability to communicate with people is poor.

At the time when the child becomes aware of its ability to make decisions and to influence others, disturbance often takes the form of temper tantrums, or of terror and panic attacks when the child feels overwhelmed by its own failures. Nightmares and periods of withdrawal into phantasy may be expressions of the child's difficulties.

As the child gets older behaviour disorders become more common. At school there may be complaints of bullying, disobedience and truancy and at home there may be defiance and disobedience.

When the child resorts to destructive or delinquent behaviour parents may become particularly worried and exasperated.

A child's pattern of disturbed behaviour may of course persist beyond the phase of development when it first appeared. Children learn whether crying, whining, bullying or temper-tantrums best solve their problems, and characteristic patterns of interaction develop in the families of disturbed children.

The Family

Even if it is too soon to hope that in the future adult mental illness will be prevented by the treatment of maladjusted children, it is necessary and helpful to break the vicious circle which results when the parents feel unable to handle the difficult situation created by the child's disturbed behaviour. The parents feel guilty, they experience mounting anxiety and helplessness and fear of criticism by friends and relatives. The child in turn reacts to the tension at home by becoming more disturbed. It is not usually the severity of the child's disturbance, but the parents' feeling of inadequacy that first causes psychiatric help to be sought.

The psychiatrist takes the whole family situation into account when treating children. Not only the child's behaviour but the mother's feelings about him are investigated. During treatment a better understanding of the child's problems is often acquired by the parents and the child sometimes becomes sufficiently self-confident and adaptable to remain well, even if upsets occur in the family.

Admission to hospital, or even to a child guidance clinic as an out-patient, creates considerable conflict in the parents. It appears to them to be an admission of failure to have to seek help, and often they feel guilty and responsible for the child's illness. The hospital staff is sometimes treated with resentment and hostility as a result of this, and the hospital is criticized. The parents of a mentally ill child require as much sympathy, help and understanding as does the patient.

The doctor always obtains a history from the parents and encourages them to speak freely before asking detailed questions. Later the psychiatric social worker gives the parents the help they require and interprets to them the approach of the psychiatrist and the hospital. She also helps the parents to understand their fears and to overcome their mistrust of the hospital and in particular of the nursing staff. Gradually they realize that their own failure to help the child is not interpreted as incompetence and that the nurses are not competing with them for the child's love and affection.

Treatment of the Disturbed Child

Admission to hospital becomes necessary when a crisis occurs in the home and parents and child need a rest from each other, or when insufficient information is available from the parents and additional information is required from hospital staff who are able, by close observation, to assist in the assessment of the child's problem. The child is not always clearly aware of the reasons for admission to hospital. He may believe admission to be punishment for past misdeeds and resent the hospital and its staff. On the other hand, he may have very clear ideas about the help he would like but his ideas may not quite coincide with those of his parents. He may wish for some magic to remove his troublesome baby sister, for example, or for some medicine which might make him a good boy or for some operation which might change him into the kind of child his parents would prefer—into a girl for example or into a bright boy who is good at school.

It is important that the child's story should be listened to and his point of view respected if treatment is to be effective. If the child believes that doctor and nurses only listen to the mother's side of the story he may not find it easy to express his own problem and difficulties. The general attitude should convey to the child that the staff are on his side and eager to understand how he feels.

Though children are often admitted after considerable tension at home, separation from the parents is nevertheless frequently traumatic. Homesickness and a period of grief and distress are very common during the early days of hospitalization.

The hospital ward must provide a warm, friendly, harmonious background. Daily routine should be normal for the child's age and level of development.

Very young children can establish successful relationships with only a few individuals and all disturbed children have difficulties in making contact with many people at one time. A stable nursing staff is therefore required. Whenever possible the child should have one special nurse whom he can consider to be his own.

The routine must be flexible, according to the child's age and degree of illness, yet it must be sufficiently fixed to give him a sense of security.

The routine of children's wards must, of necessity, be different from that of adult wards because the normal pattern of activity for children is totally different.

The fixed points in a child's day, as in the adult's day, are meal-times. While the adult's day has a pattern of work and leisure, the child's day has a pattern of school and play. Bedtime and bath-time have much greater significance in a child's life than in the adult's.

Small children are sticklers for precise repetition in routine. The fact that the soap is in a different place in hospital from home may greatly distress a small child.

The precise order in which dressing, washing or preparation for meals are carried out may be very important to him, just as his stories must be told with specific use of words and the bedclothes must be tucked in in a specific way.

Precise repetition of daily routine is much more important to the child than to the adult, who is usually able to cope with minor alterations from day to day even if he is mentally ill.

Over a period of time, however, the child's pattern of life changes much more than the adult's. An illness, for example, of three months occupies a relatively short space of time in an adult's life. For the small child three months may seem like an eternity. He may have difficulty in imagining the future so far ahead and therefore have difficulty in believing that he has a future life outside hospital. He may be unable to remember three months back, and therefore become more seriously detached from his home and family, than the adult does in a similar time span. To be three months older means a lot to a child in terms of knowledge gained and in terms of rights and privileges.

The organization of a children's ward should, therefore, not only be concerned with providing the framework within which the child can learn to deal with his difficulties and problems but also with the provision of an environment in which the child can grow and develop.

In the daily routine school work, music, handicraft, sports, carpentry all have a definite place in the timetable according to age. Outdoor activities must be arranged. The rest of the day can be spent in free play or games, entertainments, parties, stories or quiet reading.

The weekly routine means that each day is different from the others. Outings and visitors are planned for the week-end, different lessons take place on different days of the week. A predictable pattern emerges from the off-duty arrangements of the nursing staff and the interviews with the doctors. Children need target days for which to prepare and which divide the year into measurable periods. End of school term for example, like Christmas day or birthdays, helps to measure time. It is always helpful if some specific event is being planned—a sports day for example, an open day at school, an exhibition of paintings or the performance of a concert or play.

The activities of a children's ward should offer scope for children of all ages. Because the children are all disturbed, difficulties may arise at any time. Although when a child is upset, he may not be able to participate fully in the daily routine, the knowledge that the routine exists is of importance. He must know what he is meant to do, even if at the moment he is unable to comply. If there is nothing for him to do boredom sets in and increases the disturbance.

Each group of children may be interested in different pursuits and each nurse should use her own ideas and resourcefulness. One of the few general rules is always to take part in the children's activities. If the nurse is an uninterested, detached observer, she finds it very difficult to influence the children's activities. If she participates, she can suggest changes if the group becomes too wild or control over the game is lost, or if she feels that boredom might disrupt the group.

It is a good plan for the nurse always to have one or two new ideas up her sleeve when she is looking after children. When all are happy the children suggest their own activities. When interest flags it is useful to introduce something new and exciting, quickly and without delay.

The general attitude and approach to disturbed children is determined by the fact that the disturbance is considered to be a symptom of illness, not a sign of wickedness. All the staff are able to treat the child's behaviour with tolerance if they understand that he is unhappy, perhaps frightened, and very much in need of love. When children are mentally ill very few rules of behaviour can be laid down or enforced. This does not mean that antisocial behaviour should be encouraged. On the contrary, the nursing staff should try to make clear to the children what are desirable standards of behaviour. They can do this by example, by encouragement, approval of appropriate behaviour, positive suggestion to the child. Nurses can make it easier for a child to behave well by making few demands. But when uncontrolled, disturbed behaviour does occur it is treated in a matter-of-fact, unemotional manner and without moral condemnation.

The Role of the Nurse

One of the duties of the nurse is the prevention of physical injury to children or staff and as far as possible the limitation of damage to property. It should be made clear that overtly antisocial acts cannot be permitted and that the child will be prevented from injuring himself or others. This may have to be done by removing the child bodily and if necessary more than one nurse must be available. There is no need for anger to be shown. As soon as possible the nurse must convince the child that her love is not affected. No humiliation of the child should be involved and peace is re-established automatically once the disturbance is over, without any need for the child to 'lose face'.

Children who have lacked love and approval often find it difficult to believe that they really are accepted by the nurses. For a little while they enjoy the approval they receive and behave very well. Gradually they feel compelled to test the sincerity of the staff and their behaviour becomes worse, as if to provoke hostility and force the staff to show their hand. Continued friendliness drives the child to further experimentation.

Gradually he becomes anxious and frightened, wondering how far he can go, and eventually forces the issue with a full-blown outburst of aggression.

Calm, quiet nursing staff, who remain in control of the situation, usually reassure him sufficiently for him to settle down in the ward.

Behaviour which may be acceptable because a child is severely disturbed may be imitated by other children who are well enough to go home soon, and who may have to learn to submit to the usual social sanctions. This raises the question of possible punishment. Punishment may be necessary as the child recovers. It is often demanded by the child whose sense of justice may be the best guide when it is difficult to differentiate between naughtiness and illness. No physical punishment can ever be used in hospital. Punishment in the form of exclusion from some activity may satisfy the demand for justice without causing resentment.

Some disturbed children are too frightened and too timid to be naughty at all. A certain amount of defiance, breaking of rules and naughtiness may be the first and very welcome sign of improvement. It would be very wrong if punishment were to frighten such a child back into submission. One of the most difficult tasks is to know what any particular action means to the child and when ordinary social standards should be applied in judging behaviour.

Normally children learn to forego immediate gratification of their wishes and to accept the restrictions of society, in order to retain the love, affection and approval of the person whose approval and love is valued. Usually the close tie with the mother helps the child to learn social codes and to deal satisfactorily with all the frustrations and emotional turmoils which occur in the process. When the emotional upheaval is too great and terrifying, or when the child has not been able to form a close emotional bond with an adult, he may fail to adapt in the normal way.

A child who lacks love and affection can progress only when he succeeds in forming a close relationship with somebody. If the nurse becomes the person whose love and approval is valued by the child, it is sufficient for her to make her standards known. The child will soon learn to conform. Unlimited love and affection are needed by most disturbed children. But the nurse who has successfully become the object of attachment must be careful not to disappoint the child, who would feel badly let down if 'his nurse' were suddenly moved from the ward. Gradual detachment and displacement of affection to another person may be helped by the doctor if it is planned ahead.

Innumerable problems inevitably arise when dealing with emotionally disturbed children. Each difficulty must be overcome as it arises, no general rules can be given, each nurse must develop sufficient self-confidence to make decisions as and when they become necessary. Each must become aware of her own ability to prevent a group of children from becoming uncontrolled. Each must discover for herself how and when it is safe to make demands on children and when to refrain. It is useful to remember how difficult it is to enforce an order given to a child. It is much better not to give it at all if it cannot be enforced. It is usually possible to suggest an activity rather than order it. If the suggestion is not taken it does not damage the prestige of the nurse. 'Go and have a bath' is a command which may have to be carried out by force if it is not obeyed, but 'How about having a bath?', 'I'll turn your bath water on', or 'It is now bath time', will probably have the desired effect. If it does not, the idea of the bath can be dropped and nobody is the loser.

Many orders given to children and many prohibitions are really unnecessary. The nurse would do well always to hesitate before saying 'Don't', and to decide if she really means to be obeyed. If so, she must be prepared to enforce conformity. If it is not really essential, she might as well refrain from forbidding the action.

If the nurse is to feel free to make her own spontaneous decisions in case of difficulty she must feel secure in her relationship to the rest of the staff. Ward morale in a children's ward requires constant attention. Arguments about children in front of other children undermine confidence and authority. Children learn to exploit differences of opinion among the staff, and become insecure. All staff concerned with the treatment of the child should periodically discuss his progress and try to assess the part each one plays in treatment. Harmony among the staff is as important a factor in the treatment of disturbed children as is harmony in the home in the prevention of maladjustment.

The nursing care of disturbed adolescents has many factors in common with the care of adults, and many with the care of children.

Adolescents do not get on very well in adult wards. When there is only one young person among adults he tends to get pampered and spoilt at first and later becomes a nuisance to the older patients who become irritated by the very behaviour they first encouraged.

When young people get together in a group they tend to be noisy, untidy and boisterous and are disliked by older patients. It is not easy either, to care for adolescents in children's wards. If they behave responsibly they tend to be treated too much like staff substitutes. If they are very disturbed their influence on smaller children can become disruptive and bullying can become a problem.

Special wards for adolescent boys and girls can be so organized that their varied needs are met.

Children are officially allowed to leave school at the age of 15 but many stay on at school and take school-leaving examinations. Psychiatric illness should not interfere with their educational opportunity.

If good educational facilities are provided for those still at school, some of those who have already left may become interested in further education. For those who have started work some occupational training can be of great value.

Adolescence is a time when young people are faced with problems of adjustment to work. The activities of the ward should, therefore, include school, occupational training and work for those who need it.

Adolescent leisure activities include sport, dancing and pop music but not all young people want to indulge in these activities all the time. For many adolescents the period in hospital can provide the opportunity to discover the wide range of leisure pursuits available and their own special aptitude and interest.

Preoccupation with clothes and personal appearance is common among young people. Nurses sharing this interest can help to develop self-respect and self-reliance. Hairdressing and dressmaking can be time consuming activities in adolescent wards.

Of course, young people want to look their best, not to gain approval from the staff, but to be attractive to members of the opposite sex. Girls and boys need the opportunity to meet, and they need help in making friends with each other. There are periods of great elation when friendships develop and great tragedy when they go wrong. The support of their group and of sympathetic staff is necessary in their learning experiences.

Adolescents gain perhaps more than patients in any other age group from association with each other. Interests of any one member of the group may readily be taken up by others; together they can experiment with art, music, carpentry or engineering. In discussion with each other, they can test the validity of their opinions and explore ideas and beliefs. With each other's support they can reveal their hostility to their parents, their struggle with authority and their continuing need for dependence. They can help each other to make a more realistic choice of a career than they might do alone.

Relationships with nursing staff depend largely on the nurse's age. Because some nurses are very near in age to adolescent patients they find it difficult to accept the patient's disturbed behaviour. It requires maturity to be able to understand the rebelliousness of young people without moral judgement. Many adolescent patients have experienced so much condemnation and punishment before admission that they expect to be rejected by the staff in the hospital, and it is unfortunate if their experience is repeated. The provision of control and safe limits to the patient's behaviour is necessary, without re-enforcing the patient's pattern of antisocial behaviour and punishment. If in-patient treatment of adolescent patients is successful, it is in some measure due to the fact that some nurses succeed in becoming accepted members of the adolescent group and can act as models for better-adjusted behaviour. Some members of staff, because they care about the adolescent patient and understand his problems, succeed in providing adult standards and requirements which the patient can accept. As the patient grows up and matures and learns, in the hospital community, to become tolerant of other people's behaviour he may become capable of better understanding of his own parents when he leaves.

BOOKS FOR FURTHER READING

B. Bettelheim. (1965) *Love is not Enough*. Collier, New York.

M. Burn. (1956) *Mr. Lyward's Answer*. Hamish Hamilton, London.

D. Miller. (1964) *Growth to Freedom*. Tavistock, London.

CHAPTER 13

The Nursing of Old People

An overwhelming majority of the patients in psychiatric hospitals at present are old people and a very large proportion of newly admitted patients are over sixty years of age. Although the patients suffer from a wide variety of mental disorders, it is useful to examine to what extent the nursing problems are determined by old age, rather than by the disorder. There are, broadly speaking, three groups of older patients.

1. Those whose mental illnesses resemble disorders occurring in young people, but who happen to be getting on in years. Many of these patients, e.g. those suffering from depressive illnesses, have had previous attacks and may have been in hospital before.

2. Those whose mental illness is an accompaniment of old age. Senile dementia is an example of the disorders of this group.

3. Patients who have spent many years in psychiatric hospitals and who have grown old there. Some schizophrenic patients, for instance, may have been admitted at the age of twenty and may still be in hospital at the age of sixty-five or seventy. This last group includes some patients who have partly recovered from the illness which has occasioned their admission but who had no home to which to go when their discharge from hospital would have been possible. Others may have had recurrent attacks of mental illness, returned home slightly less efficient after each attack, and have finally remained in

hospital when, owing to their own increasing age, the family no longer found it possible to shoulder the burden of caring for an old and troublesome patient.

THE REACTIONS OF OLD PEOPLE

The specific care of each patient depends partly on the nature of his illness, partly on the prospect he has of being discharged. To a large extent it is determined by age alone, and here it is proposed to examine the problems of nursing old people in psychiatric hospitals irrespective of the illness from which they suffer.

All who are sick and admitted to hospital react to their dependence on nurses and doctors in a manner which is in some way determined by their previous experience of similar relationships. Most adult patients, for instance, react to the nurse in a similar way to that in which, many years before, they treated their mother who provided food, care and comfort. According to the patient's own previous pattern he treats the nurse, the 'mother figure', with love and gratitude, with adulation, or with hate and resentment. Old people occasionally adopt the attitude of previous childish dependence. More often, however, they do not allow themselves to accept this position and instead, in the manner of some adolescents, they endeavour to prove their independence, showing militant resentment towards those whose authority they are unwilling to accept.

Normally, particularly in the case of physically ill patients, the nurse can exploit the phase when the patient accepts dependence, use it to build up prestige and will be grateful for the patient's non-critical submission to treatment. Nevertheless, the nurse should be aware of the abnormal characteristics of this phase and detect the first signs of recovery, when the patient assumes his role of independence and begins to become more critical and impatient. In the case of old people, complete dependence is rare and it would perhaps be a bad thing if it occurred. Perhaps the patient's desperate attempt to cling to independence, to assert it and to resist letting himself go, represents the basis on which to build when the nurse tries to help him to rehabilitate in preparation for discharge. But the immediate effect is that old people are difficult to nurse. They find it necessary to assert their independence, as if, otherwise, their claim to greater wisdom and experience might be overlooked. Far from manifesting uncritical acceptance of the nurse's endeavour to help, old people are constantly finding fault and reminding her of her shortcomings. Far from accepting authority in medical matters, old patients are rebelliously antagonistic to all efforts on their behalf. The patient resents being dependent, and particularly being dependent on a young person, someone the age of his granddaughter.

This relationship might create difficulties if, in her turn, the nurse showed resentment and hostility or if she were to react by adopting a patronizing attitude to the old patient. These attitudes are quite commonly found in the patient's own family relationships. The daughter, finding the patient rather difficult to manage, becomes hostile and refuses to help or begins to feel ashamed of her elderly relative and becomes patronizing, thereby aggravating already strained relationships. Nurses only too frequently adopt a condescending attitude to elderly patients. Sometimes they show it in their dealings with the patients, sometimes it emerges only in talking about them. It is of utmost importance for the nurse, if she wishes to make a success of her task, to take herself in hand when she discovers such an attitude in herself. Old people are entitled to regard and esteem by virtue of their superior age alone. To the patient, nurses may be mere children, people whom he considers young, irresponsible and inexperienced. He is paying the nurse a great compliment by entrusting her with his welfare.

Habits established over a period of a lifetime are difficult to change, and, with advancing years, it becomes more difficult to learn new ones. To a young patient, it may not matter greatly that meals in hospital are served at a different time from the one to which he is used; to the older one this may be a continued source of irritation. Hospital routine obviously differs in many respects from the régime to which each patient is accustomed. It cannot always be made to suit the individual patient's wishes. By making hospital routine fairly constant and rigid the patient may in time accept it. This is a difficult task for the patient and his difficulty should be appreciated. On discharge, he has to make new adjustments in many ways as difficult as the first one. With patience and understanding he can be assisted in adapting himself, but, wherever possible, he should be spared the effort of doing so. Many of the patient's habits could easily be carried over into hospital life if a little effort were made to adapt hospital routine to the patient. Unless his behaviour is decidedly harmful to himself or others, there is no reason why he should not continue to behave in the way he has always done. He is very unlikely, for example, to change his table manners, or his preferences for certain articles of food. Some nurses, while appreciating the patient's difficulties, show their condescension by talking about 'letting the patient have his little ways'. These may be 'little' to the nurse but the irritation caused by unnecessary interference may assume mountainous dimensions in the view of those who are ill, and may seriously impede the nurse in essential nursing matters.

The Physical Requirements of the Old

The old person's physical health must be considered when the nursing care or routine of the ward is planned. Old people find stairs very difficult to manage. They become breathless when climbing upstairs, may easily stumble and fall when coming downstairs and are fatigued if required to climb stairs several times a day. This presents a major problem to the planning of psychiatric hospitals and to the allocation of existing wards. Ground floors would be so much more suitable for almost all patients that it is difficult to allocate priorities. Stairs may make it difficult for older patients to participate fully in those social and occupational events which take place away from the wards and may seriously interfere with their use of the garden and enjoyment of fresh air. Those patients who could move about were it not for the stairs, but who are compelled to remain in the ward if stairs have to be negotiated, should be placed in ground-floor wards. Those who are able to go upstairs should be given plenty of time, encouraged to walk slowly and assisted when necessary. A nurse should always be below patients on the stairs. Hand-rails should be provided and stairs kept in good repair. Nurses should report at once when a step is faulty or when patients experience difficulty with sloping steps, or steps which are not clearly visible. Good lighting on staircases is essential and nothing must be left lying about on the treads.

Within the ward nurses should be constantly on the lookout for anything that may contribute to accidents. Highly polished floors are dangerous and the use of small rugs should be avoided. Old patients who cannot lift their feet too well are liable to stumble and fall. Needless to say, the floor under a rug should never be polished. Furniture should be firm and fairly heavy. Patients are not likely themselves to move furniture, so that its weight is not a disadvantage. Heavy furniture allows patients to lean on it. Old people often use the furniture for support when they move or when they get tired, and it would be highly dangerous were it to give way. Any broken furniture should be instantly repaired, or at least moved out of the way. The process of sitting down or of getting up may be most cumbersome for an old person and chairs must give full support when the patient tries to raise himself. High seats and upright backs are on the whole more comfortable for old people than chairs with low seats and reclining backs.

Fire guards are essential where old people are being nursed. The elderly should never climb a ladder or even stand on a chair in order to reach their belongings. Bathrooms are places of potential danger. Many old people cannot manage to get in and out of a bath-tub unaided and for this reason some old people have not had a bath for a considerable time prior to admission. The patient may resist when a bath is suggested in hospital and the nurse may have to reassure the patient that she will give all the help required. Even with help, however, bathing may be a difficult procedure. A hand-rail on the bath is a help and some modern baths are fitted with one, but old-fashioned baths with very high sides are a problem. The bath should be accessible from both sides. It may be helpful to put a mat into the bath to prevent slipping. Baths of better design, particularly for elderly patients, are needed in many psychiatric hospitals.

Old people require assistance with washing and dressing. It may become very difficult for them to fasten garments at the back and almost impossible to put on socks and stockings. Some patients cannot tie up shoelaces because they cannot bend down without losing their balance or feeling giddy, and they cannot raise the leg high enough to place it on a chair. For the same reason old patients have difficulties in washing their feet and cutting toenails. All old people should be provided with the services of a chiropodist. It is also tiring for many old patients to raise their arms to brush and comb the hair and, unless assistance is given, the hair may then not receive enough care.

Psychiatric patients, when they are old, do not differ from other old people in the amount of assistance they require, but they differ in their attitude to those who are able and willing to give help. They are often unable or unwilling to ask for help and accept it grudgingly when it is offered. Much depends on the nurse's approach. If she does not wait to be asked but offers help, anticipating the patient's needs, making it appear that the patient is doing the nurse a favour by allowing her to help, she may succeed. She must, however, refrain from doing too much for the patient. Old people should remain active to the limit of their capability.

OCCUPATIONS FOR OLD PEOPLE

It is generally agreed that old people are much happier and healthier if they continue to work and have some interest. Those who continue to work beyond their normal retiring age usually appreciate the fact that they are still able to be useful members of the community, independent by earning at least a small amount of money. After retirement, those with many and varied interests are a great deal more contented than people whose only interest has been in their work. The happiest old people are those who have begun to take up new hobbies before retirement and who have looked forward to the day when they would be able to devote more time to the occupations they enjoy.

Old people are slower in their actions than are the young, and there are many things they cannot do at all. They should never be expected to lift heavy objects and they must be protected from the risk of physical injury, but if any job can be found within their physical capacity they should be allowed and encouraged to do it. There are many jobs in psychiatric hospitals which old patients can do quite as well as young ones. They can clean the wards, sweep, dust, polish furniture and brass, but not of course scrub floors. They can prepare meals, wash up and lay tables. According to ability and previous experience they may sew or help in the laundry. Anyone skilled in these crafts can make rugs, knit, embroider cushions or make toys.

It is desirable that old people should work among others of their own age, not in competition with younger and stronger patients. Arrangements may have to be made for more frequent rest pauses or for sitting down where others could be expected to stand. No patient should work beyond the point of fatigue. Half-day occupation is probably enough for old people, because they need more time than others for getting to the place of work and take longer for all their other activities. The slower tempo of old people is one of the main reasons why it is desirable not to mix with young ones in the wards. The routine should be specially designed to take into account their slow movements and their need for more time and more help with everything they do.

Usually old people do not mind rising early. They are often awake from early hours, and prefer to get up. They should be allowed to take their time over dressing and washing and not be rushed. They cannot be expected to be well groomed if they are not allowed enough time. It is much better for the patient to dress slowly than for him to be dressed by a nurse. Plenty of time should be allowed for meals, which should be peaceful, leisurely occasions, looked forward to and enjoyed by all. The patient requires a rest period during the day, probably after lunch, and ample time must be allowed for exercise in the garden, since this entails the changing of shoes and putting on of overcoats and warm clothing.

ENTERTAINMENT

Evening entertainments are better enjoyed by the old people if they are among themselves, although they appreciate an occasional chance of watching the young ones at a dance. It may be possible to develop new interests, but it takes a long time and the new activity must be started and well established by somebody before it is taken up by those who have never done it before. It is a common experience that there are vogues for certain types of handicraft. One patient may be an expert at knitting bedjackets. If her efforts are suitably admired by all, particularly by the nursing staff, some other patient may decide to try. Soon there may be a third patient trying it and, before long, most patients may be knitting bedjackets. In due course, this activity is replaced by a new one, e.g. embroidery or production of shopping bags, each activity being started and spread in the same manner. Interest in entertainments develops in a similar way. It is no use asking patients if they wish to go to a whist drive. It should be taken for granted that a few will go. Within a few weeks, more and more patients also do so.

Initiative as regards new activities often comes from the nursing staff. The nurse should sit down and play the piano, if she knows how, rather than ask if the patients would like her to, or wait until they ask her. She should be the first to sit down to a game of cards or initiate a singsong. It is unlikely that the patients would ever start without her lead.

Hearing and eyesight usually deteriorate in old age. Many of the activities taking place in hospital cannot be enjoyed by old patients because they are unable to follow clearly what is happening. Plays on the stage are often wasted on them, they cannot understand the jokes and find other people's hilarity irritating. Radio and television can be enjoyed only if the patient can adjust the set to his own liking, he cannot listen in a group or watch television from the back of the room. In handicrafts he may be able to carry out large movements and distinguish a large pattern, but he may become clumsy and inaccurate if he is asked to do fine work. It should be possible to predict whether a patient is likely to enjoy a particular entertainment and he should not be put into a position where it is brought home to him that his senses are failing and that he is falling off in efficiency.

Failing eyesight and defective hearing may give rise to many misunderstandings between patients and staff. The patient may not understand what is said to him and do the opposite to what was asked. He may think he understood and accuse the nurse of mis-stating the truth. He may know that nurses are speaking, but if he does not hear clearly he may become suspicious and irritable and feel that people are talking about him.

He may become forgetful and mislay his belongings, and then accuse others of having taken them; or he may tell jokes or stories over and over again, having forgotten that he has previously told them. Conversation between old people frequently amounts to two monologues, each one pursuing his own thoughts and paying little attention to the other. In conversation with old patients the nurse should try to follow their thoughts, and, if she wants to make herself understood, to speak in such a way that the patient really attends to her.

HEALTH

The physical health of all old patients must be carefully watched. Coughs should be taken notice of early in order to prevent the development of chronic bronchitis; varicose veins and ulcers should receive attention. The nurse must ensure that each patient receives and takes an adequate, balanced diet and that bowel action is regular. In old men, it is necessary to ensure that the bladder is properly emptied and the possibility of enlargement of the prostate should be borne in mind and any early symptoms reported.

Most old people sleep badly and many require some

form of sedation. With well-regulated activity during the day, the patients should succeed in getting a few hours' sleep at night. Old people do not sleep very deeply and if they sleep in dormitories they disturb each other. Most doctors agree that mild sedation is to be preferred to restless nights and the nurse should observe the effect which the sedative has on the patient in order to ensure that the right kind of drug is prescribed. Restlessness at night is sometimes due to frequency of micturition, and this should be noticed by the night nurse. Sometimes confusion and restlessness at night is the first indication of heart failure. A careful report by the night nurse may lead to earlier diagnosis of heart trouble than would otherwise be possible.

So far, problems affecting all old people irrespective of their illness have been discussed. A few words must now be said about special aspects of various forms of mental disorder in old age.

Of the three groups of patients, those who are most in need of help are those who are newly admitted. Almost invariably, admission was preceded by a series of crises of increasing severity. Admission to a psychiatric hospital is feared by patients and relatives and resorted to only when no other action is possible. By the time this happens, personal relationships at home have reached breaking point, and are made even worse by the sense of failure and feelings of guilt experienced by those who are ultimately responsible for initiating admission. Young people are so frequently reminded of their responsibility towards the older generation, and so often blamed for the plight of old people, that many will go to any extreme in trying to preserve their aged relative from what appears to them the terrible fate of admission to a psychiatric hospital. The relatives require all the reassurance they can be given that their difficulties are appreciated and they should receive all possible reassurance in the struggle with their feelings of guilt and shame. It is often simpler for strangers than for relatives to deal with difficult behaviour in the elderly.

Relatives should be helped to realize that admission to a psychiatric hospital, however late in life, need not be final and that their continued interest is essential if the patient is to return to them after recovery. Often the psychiatric social worker has to undertake the task of maintaining the relatives' interest in the patient and of giving the former enough support to make them willing and able to take the patient back.

Old patients who are newly admitted are often in need of help but reject this with all their might. These are the patients who are often physically below par, under-nourished because, living alone, they have been unable to cater for themselves and have not asked for help or have refused it. They may have neglected their appearance for some time, and may be dirty, badly clothed and unkempt. They are often very lonely people. As age advances, many friends die, others live too far away to maintain contacts and it is difficult to make new ones. Opportunity does not often arise of meeting new people, and, if it does, the patient may have made himself sufficiently disagreeable to frighten away other possible contacts. The fewer the patient's interests and hobbies, the more difficult it is for him to find satisfaction. Admission to hospital means a complete change in the patient's life to which he may find it very difficult to submit.

The aim in nursing the patient must be to help him to leave hospital in the shortest possible time, better equipped to deal with the problems of old age, which he will inevitably have to face. The nurse can help to do this if she understands as fully as possible just where the patient's particular problems lie, and resists adopting towards him an attitude which might repeat the old situation. While helping the patient to regain better physical health, a routine is established which he should be able to follow after discharge. He is helped to regain self-confidence and self-respect by becoming useful within the hospital and the way is paved for some occupation to be pursued after discharge. Occupational therapy must therefore take a form which can be continued in the patient's own home. If he can learn to make something with which he might earn a little money, all the better.

While the patient is in hospital he is helped to make friends. This is comparatively easy in hospital where there are fellow sufferers. After discharge, he may be able to maintain his newly formed friendships by joining clubs either of former patients or other old people's clubs. During his stay in hospital he has been helped to develop new interests and to enjoy leisure-time activities of the kind offered by many clubs. While in hospital he should be encouraged to maintain his interest in the outside world, by talking with visitors about life outside, by conversation with nurses and by keeping directly in touch with the outside world. Old patients should be taken out for walks and should do shopping outside the hospital, so that they can manage traffic, deal with money and use public transport. If they are kept too long away from the hustle of the street they find it terribly difficult to go back. Coach trips and outings are of value, but even more important are such simple activities as crossing the road, paying for bus tickets, handling the money to pay for a cup of tea.

Meanwhile, with help, the patient's relatives examine more dispassionately their own difficulties. They realize to what extent mental illness was responsible for the patient's difficult behaviour. They observe how nurses and doctors handle the situation and how the patient responds. Gradually, first at week-ends, they prepare to take the patient back for short periods and eventually accept full responsibility for looking after a difficult old person, having the reassuring knowledge that the hospital is always willing to give help whenever it is required.

It is not always possible to discharge the patient home, but active interest on the part of relatives helps, even if he has to remain permanently in hospital or be transferred to a home.

In many respects old age is much less difficult for the patient who has grown old in hospital. For him no change is involved. He is generally in better physical health, well cared for, and in many ways leads a fuller life than many old people normally do. He is not lonely and no retirement problems arise. His job in the hospital can go on indefinitely as long as he can manage it. He has had time to develop many interests because the programme of social events in hospital is quite extensive. Unless the patient is suffering from dementia, or has been allowed to become passive and helpless, the main nursing task is to make each patient's life as rich and useful as his own health and hospital conditions allow.

The nursing care of demented patients requires special skills which will be referred to in Chapter 14.

BOOKS FOR FURTHER READING

A. N. Exton Smith, D. Norton and R. McLaren. (1962) *An Investigation of Geriatric Nursing Problems in Hospital.* The National Corporation for the Care of Old People, London.

D. Norton. (1967) *Hospitals of the Long-Stay Patient.* Pergamon, Oxford.

F. Post. (1965) *The Clinical Psychiatry of Late Life.* Pergamon, Oxford.

B. Robb. (1967) *Sans Everything.* Nelson, London.

CHAPTER 14

Habit Training and Rehabilitation

It is the aim of all nursing to prepare the patient as rapidly as possible for discharge, or, if this cannot be achieved, to help the patient to remain active within the hospital and ambulant as long as can be managed.

There are at present many patients in psychiatric hospitals who, because in the past this aim was not so clearly recognized, have become helpless and bedridden and whose habits have deteriorated to such an extent that they are incontinent, unable to attend to their physical needs and unable also to respond to any form of emotional or social stimulation. In recent years, many enthusiastic workers in psychiatric hospitals have made it their business to rehabilitate these patients, and by consistent effort have in many cases achieved successes well beyond their own expectations.

In future it will be the nurses' task never to allow patients to deteriorate to the degree to which they did in the past. It will be their function to train patients who cannot improve or recover in such a way that they will at least be able to attend to feeding, elimination and personal hygiene. This, in the case of demented patients, can be achieved only if all these actions are carried out habitually, requiring no choice, decision or thought.

The Purpose of Habits

Habits are acquired by practice. When a habit is

satisfactorily established the action is performed without thought, in precisely the same manner on each occasion. In ordinary life many things are done habitually, leaving freedom for conscious effort to be devoted to more important and complex matters. Little thought is given, for instance, to dressing or brushing of the teeth. Table manners are a matter of habit; there is no need to think about which hand to use for knife or fork. Such skills as writing or typing are also habits. Habits are useful, because they save much effort. If, however, habitual actions are impeded, they may be easily discarded and a new pattern of behaviour deliberately chosen. If, for example, a finger is bandaged this results in consciousness of the mechanism of writing; in such an instance thought is given to the performance of the action by holding the pen differently or by trying to use the other hand. Or, without troubling much about it, it may be possible to postpone writing altogether, or to dictate letters to someone else. Although it may be a habit to rise at a certain time, put on clothes in a certain order, sit on a particular chair, eat breakfast before starting the day's work, it is nevertheless easy to alter this routine on holiday or on a visit to someone else's house.

HABIT TRAINING OF LONG-TERM PATIENTS

When patients are nursed back to health and prepared for successful adaptation to different circumstances, constant guard must be kept against habits becoming too fixed. Although a firm adherence to ward routine is comforting to many patients, giving them the sense of security they need, change and variety are carefully introduced to enable them to practise and enjoy an increasing ability to adapt to new situations.

When, however, the decision has been made that a patient cannot be discharged and must spend the rest of his life in hospital, a mode of life which is best suited for him within the hospital must be planned. By careful training, and by following an invariable routine, he is helped to establish a habit pattern which will enable him as successfully as possible to manage his own life. If this training is started early enough and the patient is not allowed to become bedridden and helpless, this object is not very difficult to attain. When, however, training begins after the patient has already deteriorated beyond the stage it is hoped to maintain, the task is formidable and calls for the utmost skill and ingenuity. Many hospitals have developed successful schemes of habit training, most of which are variations of the one here outlined.

The Use of Groups

It is useful to form small groups of patients, each in charge of one nurse. The patients should all be capable of approximately the same amount of activity. The more helpless and deteriorated the patients, the smaller the group which one nurse can successfully supervise. The nurse is responsible for devising a daily routine which she should carry out without the slightest variation. Gradually, one by one, the patients acquire the habits which the nurse is trying to teach. The most helpless patients, hitherto bedridden and incontinent, start by getting out of bed, sitting in a chair and being placed on a commode chair at the same time every day. Washing, cleaning of teeth, dressing and undressing and eating are at first the only activities.

For each patient the same thing is done at precisely the same moment every day. At first the nurse helps a great deal and has to attend to the patients in rotation. Gradually she will encourage each patient to do an occasional move for himself. She proceeds in exactly the same way as she would teach a baby to do things for himself. When feeding the patient, the nurse may use one spoon while the patient uses another one, and every attempt the patient makes to put a spoonful of food into his mouth is applauded. When dressing, the patient can try to do up his own buttons; when washing he can try to wipe his own face. Every sign of learning, every success, must be rewarded by evidence of genuine pleasure on the part of the nurse.

While patients are very helpless the group cannot be fully occupied through the day. Possibly only one hour in every four can be actively used at first; during the rest of the day the patient, for the time being, may continue to be inactive. During training patients receive intensive care. The routine is planned in minute detail, and precisely the same series of actions performed on each occasion.

The patient's activity is gradually increased until he is occupied for most of the day. It may become possible by degrees to give attention to several patients simultaneously, each patient performing the same action in the same manner, at the same time. A patient able to take initiative may eventually assume leadership of the group.

As the patients improve, widen their scope and become more active and more able to attend to their own needs, they cease to form a homogeneous group. Some progress faster than others, others may require almost as much help as formerly. Some reorganization of groups may become necessary. It depends on the ability and understanding of the nursing staff concerned whether one nurse continues to teach the same tasks to successive groups of patients, and patients graduate from her group to more advanced ones as they progress, or whether each nurse aims to develop the activities of her own group through all its stages. Her ultimate goal is the full-time useful employment within the hospital of most of her patients. Some patients may be left behind to join less advanced groups and she may take into her own group those who were left behind by those more advanced. The success of the scheme depends entirely on the reliability of the nursing staff and on their attitude to their work.

Habit training is partly a process of establishing conditioned responses, partly an attempt at making the patients' routine simple enough to understand and remember. In a restricted space, with the same nurse always near him, the patient may be able to live a fairly normal life.

Conditioning the Patient

As in all conditioning processes, each trial aimed at eliciting a new response must follow the same pattern, and each success must be rewarded by approval. The nurse helps the patient in every way, washes him, dresses him, feeds him, takes him to the lavatory, hoping to teach him in due course to perform all this spontaneously. This is greatly helped if nursing attention is invariably accompanied by the same words on all occasions. Not too many words should be used. Very short sentences are much better than long rambling speeches which the patient cannot understand. It is useful to give a running commentary on actions which are taking place, naming the articles used each time they are handled. As the patient is dressing, the nurse may say 'Left stocking, right stocking, one shoe, another shoe', each time one of these articles is picked up.

Feeding may be given to the accompaniment of such words as 'more food', or 'another spoonful'. Eventually, the stage is reached when the patient himself carries out the action when the appropriate word is used. The manner in which it is said shows that the nurse is not really 'commanding' or 'drilling', but merely giving the cue for the action concerned. The nurse's tone of voice may be the effective stimulus, rather than the actual words used. If the tone of voice implied a command, the patient, instead of automatically responding, might remain passive.

Successful action should be rewarded, but tangible rewards, such as sweets, cannot be offered to grown-up human beings without lowering their self-esteem. Nurses have nothing other than approval to offer. Every patient, however demented, can sense approval when it is given. In order to make approval worth having, the nurse must first demonstrate to the patient her liking for him, her sympathy, warmth and interest. Some personal bond must be established. Once this has been done, evidence of pleasure and approval at every step of progress may be sufficient reward. An uninterested, bored nurse cannot possibly succeed. Just how far it is possible to rehabilitate patients who have become completely demented and passive it is difficult to say. Already, in some hospitals, patients have become sufficiently well to attend to their own personal hygiene completely unaided. Their toilet habits are now perfect, they dress and feed themselves, can carry out simple occupations successfully and join in evening entertainments. Their success is due to firmly established habits, and to remain successful there must be no interference with routine. It is to be expected that major inevitable changes, such as the appearance of new nurses or a physical illness, may lead to considerable setbacks. Small wards and pleasant surroundings contribute greatly to the success of rehabilitation programmes.

Whether or not it is possible, in some cases, to consolidate the progress by weaning patients slowly from their habits and, by introducing change, to oblige them to make an occasional decision for themselves, only time and further experience will show.

The Effect of Institutional Living

Some patients who have spent many years in psychiatric hospitals behave as if they were suffering from dementia or as if a state of chronic schizophrenic illness had rendered them dull and unresponsive. It has now been demonstrated that their condition is due not to the mental disorder which caused their admission to hospital but to the effect of institutional living itself. The terms 'hospitalization' and 'institutional neurosis' have been applied to this condition. Clearly in future it must be prevented, but patients already suffering from the ill effects of certain aspects of hospital life need help in regaining independence, initiative and zest for life.

Institutional neurosis is the effect of the patient's resignation to the conditions which prevail in some institutions. Inactivity, idleness and boredom result in a progressive withdrawal by the patient. He sits slumped in his chair or stands about in corners, and walks with a characteristic stooping gait. Facial expression is vacant and the patient takes little interest in his personal appearance. He rarely initiates action and he readily obeys orders and instructions by the staff.

Because the patient appears so inactive nurses are often unaware of his potential abilities. They act for the patient, speak for him and answer questions on his behalf. They assume that the patient does not understand, and talk about him in his presence. This authoritarian attitude of the nurses, however kind and benevolent, makes the patient even more passive and withdrawn.

Every aspect of the patient's life needs attention when a rehabilitation programme is planned. At first every encouragement is given to him to take responsibility for his own life in the ward. He can make decisions about the clothes he wears and about the choice of food. He needs facilities to attend the hairdresser; he should choose his own clothes and look after his personal belongings. Private possessions are of great importance and the patient should be encouraged to give a personal touch to his own living space, putting photographs or ornaments on his bedside table and having his own belongings on his bed. He should have a key for his own wardrobe or cupboard and keep his property safely locked away.

The patient's day should be as full as possible with a realistic programme of work and leisure. It is normal to be up and active for at least 14 hours, preferably 16 hours out of 24.

VISITORS

The most important aspect of rehabilitation concerns the patient's link with people outside the hospital. If the patient's family can be induced to take an interest this can be of utmost value, but even if relatives can no longer be traced the patient can be put in contact with members of the hospital 'league of friends' or other voluntary workers. Many hospitals have found that unrestricted visiting helps to maintain contacts. If visitors can come at any time of the day and join in the hospital activities, they can be helped to a better understanding of the patient's behaviour, and will begin to realize that they need not over-protect or fuss over him when they are alone.

Whenever possible the patient should go out with his visitors, at least to a restaurant for a cup of tea but, when it can be arranged, preferably to the visitor's house. Practice in living in the confined space of a private home and sharing in normal family life is of great help. The patient and the relatives can be encouraged to keep in touch by post. Most patients appreciate and enjoy receiving letters and postcards and can often be induced to reply.

During the time when visitors are in the hospital the nurse's help may be required to overcome embarrassment and anxiety. Relatives may become very upset if the patient does not immediately respond and may believe that their visits are not worth persevering with. They may also not realize that it is good for the patient to become involved in the problems of the family. Quite mistakenly they may believe that they should spare the patient worry and anxiety by not talking about themselves. If the nurse is available during visiting time and gets to know the patient's relatives really well she can help the visitors to establish contact more easily and keep the patient's interest alive between visits.

In order to re-establish the patient in society it is essential that he should have money to spend. On his visits home he needs to be able to pay for himself, he needs to know how much the fare home costs and how much it costs his family to visit him. If he goes to a café he should know how much it is reasonable for the shop to charge. He should be able to plan his own personal budget and know how long he must save before he can buy a suit or a coat or a pair of shoes.

WORK IN REHABILITATION PROGRAMMES

Work in hospital can in that case be of great value, provided the patient receives full industrial rate of pay for the job he does. Even if he is charged for board and lodging and consequently is left with very little pocket money, it helps the patient to regain self-esteem if he receives a full pay packet and disposes of his own money. It is humiliating and harmful to pay the patient only a few shillings when he is performing a full day's work.

Some hospitals have been able to give patients a very useful industrial training by opening up industrial workshops and receiving contracts for industrial work for which the hospital receives normal piece rates of pay. The hospital may have to employ a manager or other staff to supervise the workshop, but any profit after overheads have been paid is shared by the patients. The value of factory work, when patients come from an industrial area, lies not only in teaching the patient to do a repetitive manual task with which he may be able to earn his own living. The main purpose of it lies in getting the patient used to the atmosphere of a real place of work, away from nursing staff and doctors and reminders of sickness. The patient can develop regular work habits, submit to the directions of the foreman, learn to clock in and out, and become perceptive of unwritten rules about working speed, rest pauses, cups of tea or smoking. He can become familiar with trade union practices and work organization. Most important of all, he begins to become aware of his own significance in life and this helps to remove some of his submissiveness even in the ward setting.

For patients who are not likely to return to industrial occupations it is difficult to provide equivalent training facilities. Farms and gardens are appropriate in agricultural districts, but most psychiatric hospitals have now given up running their own farms, and for most patients farm work is inappropriate. Some hospitals have successfully moved patients from wards into flats or small cottages for a period before discharge so that they can do their own housekeeping, shopping, cleaning, cooking, entertaining friends, sewing and even carrying out small interior decorating jobs; this will all be valuable experience.

The Disabled Persons (Employment) Act of 1944 made it compulsory for certain employers to engage a percentage of registered disabled people. Those suffering from psychiatric disabilities are entitled to register as disabled and consequently may be able to find sheltered employment after leaving hospital. They may also be able to attend an Industrial Rehabilitation Unit for assessment and may be accepted for retraining in a Government course. Work in hospital if well planned and supervised can prepare the patient for these experiences.

It is not always desirable to discharge the patient from hospital and at the same time expect him to find work. Adaptation to living outside hospital is difficult enough without the additional stress of adaptation to work. Some patients need residence in hospital while they begin to work outside. Others move out of the hospital either to a hostel or to live with relatives or friends, but continue to come to the hospital to work.

Some contact with the hospital either through a social club or by visits from social workers or nurses may be necessary for a considerable period of time before the patient can finally accept complete independence.

BOOKS FOR FURTHER READING

R. Barton. (1959) *Institutional Neurosis.* Wright, Bristol.
A. L. John. (1961) *A Study of the Psychiatric Nurse.* Livingstone, Edinburgh.

CHAPTER 15

Nursing Depressed Patients

DEPRESSION

AT some time or other, everyone has felt somewhat depressed, has thought that life was just too much of an effort, hardly worth living and has felt generally 'under the weather'. Friends have days when, from their actions, appearance and words, it is evident that their mood is black. Most people have seen a friend in grief and sorrow and experienced the urge to express sympathy and yet known the helpless groping for words which would comfort or would convey their real feelings. Conventional words of condolence may then have been uttered but silence soon fell owing to an inability to console. Yet the visit paid, and even the silence, together with a sharing of his grief, gave such a friend some help and comfort.

Moods of depression do not last very long in normal, healthy people. The mentally ill patient, however, may continue to feel depressed for a very long time and the nurse must continue to comfort, well beyond the point when she actually experiences sympathetic grief with the patient.

The right thing is automatically done when a bereaved friend is visited. Anyone trying to give consolation is quiet and not noisy or boisterous. Little is said and there is no joking or looking particularly happy. No reference is made to the good things in life or to personal pleasures, and although there is intense awareness of an inability to help, the visit, which it is known will give comfort, is nevertheless paid. The slightest sign of interest on the part of the bereaved is encouraged by vividly taking up any topic he himself may broach.

In the nursing of depressed patients this is just what is being done, but for very much longer and in much more difficult circumstances. The only comfort that can be given to the patient is sympathy, interest and appreciation of his mood. The nurse continues this without ever giving the slightest sign of boredom or irritation and she responds to the slightest evidence of the depression lifting.

THE SYMPTOMS OF DEPRESSION

The feeling of hopelessness, misery and despair experienced by depressed patients is easily communicated to the nurses. Gestures, facial expression, posture, all convey the patient's dejection. He may express in words his feeling of unworthiness and guilt, and experience a desire for punishment which he may even try to inflict upon himself. Voices may comment on the patient's imagined sinful behaviour and he may consider himself too wicked to be in this world, too dangerous to others to be in contact with them.

Not all depressed patients, however, experience the deep despair with which it is relatively easy to have sympathy. Some patients feel flat, apathetic and lifeless. They are unable to respond to people, their emotions are dulled and their ability to react to others diminished. Love, hate and affection mean nothing, the patient feels indifferent and the world around him seems changed.

The absence of emotion makes it more difficult for the patient to communicate his depression to others. He becomes asocial, withdrawn and lacks energy. He experiences difficulty in thinking and does not concentrate easily on what is said to him. His speech and movement become slower, his bodily functions disordered. His with-

drawal and unresponsiveness may be so complete that
he remains immobile and mute, in a condition termed
'stupor'.

It is no easy task for the nurse to give emotional
warmth and personal care to the unresponsive patient,
who yet needs interest and affection and is aware of the
emotional attitude of the nurse, but unable to respond to
it. He is not helped by being forced into activity, and
cannot benefit from contact with too many people. The
continued bodily care and personal service given by one
or possibly a few nurses may help to re-establish a little
emotional response. The nurse should be able to give
warmth, even though she does not receive any response,
and should be able to assess the patient's ability to
receive solicitude without being overwhelmed by even
greater feelings of unworthiness. On recovery many
patients comment on the fact that attention from a nurse
was desperately needed at the time of deepest depression,
but that it seemed quite impossible to make this need
known. Any nurse who is able to respond to a patient's
need for company at a time when he cannot make the
effort to ask for it, is greatly appreciated by the patient.

Health

Depression always carries the risk of suicide, and every
patient who is depressed requires the most careful nursing if suicide is to be prevented. The nurse may be the
first person to detect suicidal tendencies and has to adopt
what measures are considered best to preserve the
patient's life. A depressed patient is often physically
unwell. Constipation, loss of appetite, skin rashes and
boils may occur, and only the most careful nursing can
prevent serious deterioration in his physical condition.
Weekly weighing may give some indication of physical
health; increase in body weight often is a precursor of
recovery. Careful attention to the patient's personal
hygiene, frequent bathing and attention to the mouth

help to prevent skin and mouth infection. Exercise, plenty of fluids to drink and a diet containing an adequate amount of roughage should prevent constipation. The patient takes little interest in his personal appearance, has no initiative, no energy and all the effort to maintain his health has to be made by the nurse.

Food

Food is distasteful to the depressed patient. He lacks appetite, and often expresses delusions of being unworthy of food, or too poor to be able to afford it. He may feel that food is rotting inside him, that his bowels are blocked, or that he has no stomach; all these are delusions which give expression to his dislike of food. His feeling of fullness, flatulence or nausea makes it difficult to ensure adequate food intake. It is useless to argue. Attempts to persuade the patient to eat must be made with caution, since these may lead to discussion of the content of the delusion and may end with the patient's refusal to eat. Success depends largely on the nurse's attitude. She should convey by her manner that she is determined not to allow the patient to go without food, although she appreciates his reasons for refusal. If the nurse indicates that whatever his objections, she will find some method of giving him adequate nourishment, the patient will often prefer the way of least resistance and allow spoon-feeding, but giving no encouragement or active help in feeding himself.

SUICIDE

Depressed patients usually improve, although without physical treatment this may take a long time. With the help of electroconvulsive therapy or drugs recovery takes place more quickly. Good nursing is aimed at preventing suicide and relieving the intense suffering of the depressed patient. The nurse's approach, her attitude and general understanding assist him in his recovery. Only skilful observation, incessant vigilance and the most intimate knowledge of her patient can help her to prevent suicidal attempts. However resentful the patient may be of being kept alive the nurse must remember that depression passes. Once he has recovered, the patient may view the present problems in a different light and be grateful that he was not allowed to kill himself. As depression deepens a patient may feel increasingly desperate and may fear that he will be unable to resist the impulse to commit suicide. Such a patient may seek admission hoping that he will be prevented from carrying out any suicidal ideas he may have. He puts his life into the hands of the nursing staff and needs the sense of security gained from being under constant observation.

It is not always easy to assess how serious the patient's suicidal intentions are, but all expressions of suicidal thoughts and every gesture the patient makes to take his life should receive full attention. Suicide is the action of a person who is desperate. Suicidal attempts may be made to draw someone's attention to the patient's plight. If the patient succeeds in his cry for help and attention is paid to him he need not resort to further suicidal acts. If his attempt is ignored, or worse still ridiculed, he might be driven to more desperate action.

Sometimes a patient improves dramatically after a serious suicidal attempt. This may be because his suffering may be interpreted as atonement for the guilt he imagines himself to carry, or it may be because his relatives or friends have suddenly understood the patient's need for support. Once the patient no longer feels abandoned he can bear to be alive.

If his suicidal attempt fails to bring his relatives to his aid, the nurse has to do the best she can to stand by the patient and provide the motive for living. If, however, the nurse also fails to pay attention to the patient, he feels almost compelled to prove how serious his despair is.

Patients sometimes tell one member of the staff about suicidal thoughts, begging this person not to betray their confidence. This should never be agreed to. However convincing the patient's plea may appear, he may in fact wish his intentions to be known. If he did not want the staff to protect him he would mention his thoughts to no one. If the nurse in whom he has confided agrees to keep the knowledge secret the patient may interpret this as an invitation to go ahead with his plans.

Some psychiatric hospitals are so designed that obvious suicidal risks are minimized. Window panes are small, making it difficult for a patient to pass through them. Windows may be blocked or locked, opening six inches at the top and bottom only, and usually sufficiently far apart to make it difficult to fasten a rope on to a window frame. Staircases are so constructed that it is impossible for anyone to throw himself over a banister, and are of short flights so there is little danger of a patient throwing himself downstairs. At the top of the stairs there are either gates or open doors. If the doors are locked they are some distance from the head of the stairs. This prevents a sudden dash towards the staircase when anyone enters the ward. There are few projections to which ropes could be fixed. Lavatory chains are replaced by handles. Pipes and radiators are covered in so that it is not possible to hide any articles behind them. Lights are placed high up, close against the ceiling; fires are guarded. The most dangerous articles are kept under lock and key. The patient has no access to such places as laboratories, operating theatres and dispensaries. Such architectural devices should, however, be as inconspicuous as possible. Very obvious special precautions may convey the suggestion of suicide to patients who may otherwise not have seriously contemplated it.

Routine Precautions against Suicide

Some hospitals take routine precautions in wards in

which suicidal patients are nursed, so as to reduce the risk of suicide by any of the more usual means. The ratio of staff to patients in these wards is relatively high and the latter are under constant observation, day and night. Routine varies in different hospitals. Whatever the routine in any particular ward, it is most important that all members of the staff should be thoroughly familiar with the rules and carry them out faithfully at all times. It is relatively unimportant, for example, whether the doors of a ward are open or locked, but very important that all members of the staff should know which doors are open, which locked, and that each should be able to rely on every other member of the team to lock those doors which are meant to be closed.

Dangerous Objects

In many hospitals patients' property is listed and checked on admission and certain potentially dangerous articles are removed if a patient is known to have suicidal thoughts. Scissors, nail files and razor blades may be taken away and the patient is told that he may ask for these articles when he needs them for use. By removing them in the first instance, and only giving them out when required, the nurse is aware of the number of sharp instruments or tools in use at any time, thus ensuring that they are used only for the proper purpose.

It is advisable to look through the patient's property most carefully on admission, because drugs or razor blades can be hidden in the most inconspicuous places. Linings of pockets or handbags are obvious hiding places but patients may secrete dangerous articles in seams, in tins of talcum powder or lipstick cases, in face-cream jars or about their own persons. If all the patient's belongings are removed on admission and only returned after careful inspection some danger is avoided. The nurses know of all the articles the patient possesses and anxiety shown by him for the return of a particular object may lead to a more thorough search and often the discovery of something that has been hidden. This, of course, apart from lessening danger, gives a valuable lead to understanding the patient's state of mind.

The patient's property is examined with the full knowledge of the patient and preferably with his assistance. To most people it is distressing and embarrassing to allow strangers access to one's personal belongings. The patient is almost certainly distressed when he knows that the nurse wishes to examine his property on admission. It may, however, be reassuring to him to know that the nurses care for him sufficiently to take the necessary precautions which ensure the safekeeping of his belongings and the safety of his person.

Nurses sometimes find the task embarrassing and for that reason might tend to hurry over the procedure. Half-hearted attempts to look at the patient's belongings do nothing to alleviate distress. If the nurse fails to discover dangerous objects the patient has secreted, the patient feels less than safe with such a nurse and consequently more anxious. The patient's property can never be examined in secret and without the patient's knowledge, firstly because this would be extremely degrading to the patient, and secondly because if any dangerous articles are found this has to be fully discussed with the patient.

Some precautionary measures are possible without excessive restriction of the patient's activities.

When clothes are marked with the patient's name, belts and pyjama cords can be stitched in, shoelaces firmly secured and the most dangerous articles of clothing kept from him until more is known about him. If no torn linen is ever used in the ward, it becomes possible at once to discover when the patient is trying to tear sheets or blankets, or collect pieces of tape which could be used at some future time to make a rope.

If all beds are regularly stripped by patients and

nurses together and if lockers are regularly cleaned out, especially after visitors have left parcels, then any dangerous object the patient may try to hide is easily discovered.

If cutlery is put out only just before a meal is due to be served and if the right amount of cutlery is always laid for each patient and collected from each patient when the meal is finished, special checking of cutlery becomes unnecessary.

If breakages occur, it is helpful if the broken pieces are cleared with all possible speed and if a nurse assumes responsibility for checking that all pieces are accounted for.

It is unusual for patients who are depressed to have baths without a nurse being present. In some hospitals or in some wards, hot-water taps are removable and used only by the nurse, never being handled by patients. Bathrooms, when not in use, are kept locked, as also are kitchens, broom cupboards and sluice rooms. Patients who are acutely depressed usually enter the kitchen only if accompanied by a nurse. The patient's clothing may be kept locked up, clothes either being handed to him by a nurse or he may be allowed access to them only when accompanied. By these means the nurse knows what the patient is wearing, and at any time could give an accurate description of him if the need arose. She also knows if the patient has any money on him, and how much, since she will herself have given it to him on request. Nurses should know which patients wear glasses and notice at once if they are missing. If any patient is wearing jewellery, wedding ring or watch, this too should be known and noted. Some patients sleep with their dentures in place, a fact which must be pointed out to the night nurse.

Matches and lighters may not be allowed in the ward and the nurse lights the patient's cigarette for him. She then knows when anyone is smoking and is able to make sure that the cigarette is put out when finished and not used to light another. This reduces the risk of fire.

Smoking in bed is usually discouraged, except when the patient is in bed all day.

Poisons

All poisons, drugs and lotions are kept under lock and key and no bottles are ever taken into the ward. If a disinfectant is required for cleaning, the pail of water is brought to the store-room and the disinfectant put into the water by a nurse. Medicines are poured out in the room in which the medicine cupboard is kept, and taken into the ward one at a time. Tablets are sometimes given crushed and powders are dissolved in water, so that they cannot be hoarded. No patient ever gains access to an open drug cupboard. Cleaning materials are kept locked, because polish and cleaning powders, such as Harpic, are potentially dangerous. Sterilizing and clinical rooms are not entered by patients. Once a treatment tray is prepared, it is never left out of sight of a nurse. If any surgical procedure is carried out, one nurse is responsible for the safety of the equipment while another carries out the treatment. Temperatures are taken in the axilla, not in the mouth, bandages are sewn, not pinned, hot-water bottles are used with greatest care. Patients should never be left while any treatment is being carried out.

When patients leave the ward the nurse should always know and she should be aware of any patient's activity at any time. At meal times patients are counted, and any patient who is missing should be sought at once. It may be necessary to lock annexes during a meal.

Observation of Suicidal Patients

If these precautions are carried out in a ward in which potentially suicidal patients are nursed, they facilitate the special care and observation which is necessary when any individual patient is known to have expressed suicidal ideas. For the sake of the patient and the staff, it may be necessary to issue 'suicidal caution' in special circumstances, and to keep a particular patient under constant observation. Whenever a member of the staff becomes aware of her patient's suicidal intentions, she must immediately report this to all who are concerned in his care. One of the most efficient methods is to issue a 'caution card' which is signed by the patient's doctor and informs all staff members that the patient is to be kept under special observation. The card states the methods by which he has attempted to take his own life, the method he has threatened to use and any method he is likely to use. Any special instruction should be recorded and all nurses should sign that they fully understand the danger before taking responsibility for the patient. The nurse who is looking after him at any time should ensure that her relief is well instructed in her duties and has signed the card before handing over. In some hospitals, patients on 'suicidal caution' are always accompanied by a nurse, but if other members of the staff, e.g. occupational therapists, assume responsibility, they too should sign the card.

While a patient is on suicidal caution he should never be out of sight or out of reach of the nurse. Whether this can be achieved when the patient is up and dressed, or whether it is necessary for him to remain in bed, depends on the staff available.

It is impossible to keep a patient under constant observation without his knowing that this is being done. The nurse should therefore meet the patient's questions quite frankly, and either herself explain the procedure to him or make sure that his doctor has done this. The patient may ask the reason for the surveillance, but is then merely expecting the nurse to confirm reasons well known to him. With a little tact the nurse can usually manage to obtain from him the explanation of why he is being observed and so avoid the embarrassment of pretending not to know.

Constant observation is an extremely arduous duty.

For parts of the day it may be possible to keep the patient occupied. Games of chess, card games, reading aloud, may make his, and the nurse's life easier, but if he is really depressed he may not wish to speak or be spoken to, there may be long periods of silence and complete inactivity on his part, during which the nurse must keep herself occupied, without ever relaxing vigilance. She must not become so absorbed in any work that she will not notice the patient's every movement, yet she cannot just sit and stare at him. The patient has little to do other than to watch the staff, and any carelessness or negligence on the part of the nurse is noticed and use may be made of this knowledge at some later date.

It is often pointed out that the effect of constant observation is that the patient observes the staff more efficiently than the nurses are able to observe the patient. It may indeed be much more dangerous to carry out constant observation negligently than to relax the rules altogether. The more it is necessary to take precautions, the more resourceful must be the patient if he is to outwit the staff. The removal from him of all the usual means of committing suicide may act as a challenge to him to find new and unusual methods.

It is perhaps with this idea in mind that some hospitals have abandoned 'suicidal caution' and constant observation, and report no increase in the incidence of attempted or successful suicide. They claim that no patient would abuse the confidence and trust which the staff have placed in him. This, however, appears to some people to represent a somewhat superficial view, even if it is true that statistically the incidence of fatalities does not rise.

The nurse's trust in the patient may prevent his suicide in hospital, but may result only in an earlier discharge, followed by successful suicide. In any case, it seems hardly fair to place the responsibility on the patient, when he may have entered the hospital for protection.

Where life is at stake, statistics seem unimportant. Even a single successful suicide is unforgivable if the nurse has to admit that she has taken no steps to prevent it. It is sad if the patient succeeds in committing suicide in spite of all precautions, but to have to admit a knowledge of the patient's intentions which were then ignored would be but cold comfort to a bereaved relative, who may well feel that he could have done better himself.

When a patient in the ward makes a suicidal attempt, or when a successful suicide has occurred, widespread repercussions are usually evident among patients and staff. Nurses feel guilty at what they perceive to be a failure in their task of preserving life. They may resort to 'scapegoating' of each other, trying to attach blame to someone in an attempt to clear their own conscience. They very naturally wish to ensure that no negligence has occurred and the serious effects of it tend to magnify the event. Nurses feel despondent and depressed, and however earnestly they may try to spare the other patients' feelings, their own emotions inevitably affect ward atmosphere.

There are usually at least a few patients who share in the self-reproach and guilt feelings of the nursing staff and who believe they might have been able to prevent the tragedy had they been more observant or more ready to confide in the staff that they knew of the patient's suicidal intentions.

The general depression in the ward is often aggravated by the anxiety patients begin to feel for their own safety. Many patients become uncomfortably aware that they may find themselves unprotected should they succumb to suicidal impulses.

Free discussion of the incident often relieves anxiety far better than an attempt to maintain secrecy. Patients often put forward constructive and practical ideas how future attempts could be prevented and often suggest methods of co-operation designed to protect each other. When patients feel able to share responsibility for each other, close observation by nurses becomes less important and the restrictive aspects of supervision can be more easily relaxed.

The Importance of Teamwork

To sum up, it may be said that the nursing of suicidally depressed patients is the acid test of a good nurse and of teamwork and co-operation. Opinions differ as to the best method to be employed. Some feel that every conceivable precaution must be taken to prevent suicide. Others believe that constant observation increases rather than relieves depression, and that in order to help the patient over his depressed mood certain risks must be taken. Those who are in favour of stringent precautions point out that the reasons for depression are unconscious, not related to the present, and that good nurses can carry out constant observation without it becoming irksome to patients. Those who prefer to give the patient a maximum of freedom point to the success of their method.

All, however, are agreed that if risks are taken, this should be done deliberately and that, while calculated risks may be justifiable, negligence is not. All are agreed that it is essential for all staff to work as a team, to be fully aware of whatever rules are in operation, and to carry out any agreed procedure with a hundred per cent efficiency. With this in mind, the most stringent care has here been described. Every nurse must ensure that she is fully aware of all the rules which apply to the ward in which she is working.

BOOKS FOR FURTHER READING

E. Stengel (1964) *Suicide and Attempted Suicide*. Penguin Books, Harmondsworth.

CHAPTER 16

Care of Disturbed and Violent Patients

MOST visitors after their first tour through a psychiatric hospital express surprise at what they have seen. Some of them ask if they could be shown real patients, those who are violent, noisy or abusive. When the few noisy patients in the most disturbed wards are indicated, visitors feel cheated and presume that something is being kept from them. The popular idea of mental illness is that of violence, aggression and danger. This idea is also often expressed by new nurses who inquire about the 'dangerous patients' and ask to be instructed as to how these may be controlled and as to how thay may protect themselves from those who are violent.

The experienced nurse knows that violence is extremely rare. Impulsive behaviour sometimes occurs, but there is little real danger of physical injury to herself. She may forget, however, that her own competence, self-assurance and tactful handling of patients is a factor in preventing violence and excitement, and that this would occur much more frequently if the nursing staff were less competent, or more tactless, aggressive or insecure. The new nurse experiences fear and misgivings, and this very insecurity is communicated to the patient, who, in the presence of one inexperienced member of the staff, may become frightened. Because he is frightened he may become aggressive. It is therefore very often the new nurse who has to bear the brunt of the violent patient and who requires some reassurance and support.

Even though excitement and violence are rare and usually appear during a short phase of the illness only, the nurse should know what to do with the patient during this phase. The reasons for disturbed and violent behaviour should be investigated in order to be better able to prevent it or to calm the patient as rapidly as possible when he becomes excited.

Aggressive or violent behaviour can nearly always be traced to disturbances in the relationships between people. Aggression is not an attribute of a person, but a response to a frustrating or frightening experience. It is a feeling most people experience at some time or another.

Children often express their aggressive feelings quite openly. When they are very young they kick and scream or have temper tantrums. As they grow older they learn to express their aggression more in speech and less in action and later still, they learn to control their aggression. There are times when they give no overt indication of it at all.

In our society considerable value is attached to this process of control.

In order to succeed in controlling aggression it is necessary, in the course of growing up, to experience it openly and to practise various methods of dealing with it. Children who are made to feel guilty about their aggressive impulses may lack practice in the process of control. Eventually they may succeed in hiding their aggression from everyone, even from themselves. They may appear meek and mild, gentle and placid. Behind this appearance may lurk the fear that to feel aggressive is dangerous and that any show of aggression might get out of control.

It is possible that unconscious fear of their own aggression is to be found in nurses too. Possibly the fear many nurses express, of being attacked by a patient, is caused by anxiety that their own aggression might be aroused by a violent patient.

It is a necessary stage in the control of aggression that one should be consciously aware of its existence. Children who have never been allowed to say that they felt angry with their parents are much more likely to have difficulty with their repressed aggressive feelings, than those children who in an angry moment can safely say to their mother, I hate you'.

In psychiatric wards patients and staff sometimes have problems in controlling their aggression. In the relative safety of a psychiatric ward patients' control may give way. Aggressive behaviour may occur in patients who had previously been unaware of their aggressive impulses. This is referred to as 'acting out'. In some respects it may be helpful in the treatment of the patient that unconscious aggression should become overt by acting out. The effect of it is, however, so disturbing to the patient himself, to the other patients and to the staff, that the aim of treatment often consists in helping the patient to 'verbalize', i.e. to talk openly about the difficulties rather than to act out.

Nurses sometimes believe that it is wrong for them to experience anger or aggressive feelings. Nurses cannot, of course, 'act out' when they feel angry. If a nurse tries to hide her feeling, some of it may nevertheless manifest itself in actions; she may break things, make unnecessary noise, be rather rougher in carrying out physical treatment than she would otherwise be, forget some attention she has promised a patient or avoid altogether speaking to a patient to whom she feels aggressive. It is as necessary for nurses as it is for patients to feel free to talk about their frustrations and anger.

Sometimes it is appropriate for the nurse to tell a patient how angry she feels. More about this will be said later in Chapter 26. Failing this opportunity, open discussion with other members of the staff is necessary in order to ensure that difficult patients can be dealt with without nurses losing control over aggressive feelings.

EXCITABLE PATIENTS

Some patients suffering from mania are in a highly active and excitable state. They feel on top of the world, full of energy, able to shoulder the greatest burdens. Their self-confidence is supreme. They feel happy, are capable of quite unusual feats, have extraordinary strength and feel able to work or keep active for long periods without tiring. They are full of ideas, but ideas occur to them so rapidly that they have no time to put any of them into operation. Everything they see or hear suggests a new line of thought. The patient is delighted with his own performance.

Those who watch him know that he is badly in need of rest, food and drink, but he has no time for any of these essentials. A course of action must be planned which will enable the patient to sleep, so that he may recover from his excessive energy output. It would be desirable that he should wash, eliminate urine and faeces in the proper place, but all this means nothing to him. He cannot understand such preoccupation with what seem to him to be trivialities. He is busy with greater things and finds people slow, dull and rather annoying. He resents interference with his activities and may become most aggressive and angry if he believes that he is not getting sufficient support.

The manic patient is easily distracted and his interest can be roused and changed by a word or gesture from a nurse. Provided the nurse has the presence of mind to detect danger before it arises and to distract the patient's attention, no one need ever be hurt by a patient suffering from mania.

Sympathy with the patient's feelings is essential. His anger when frustrated is very similar to the annoyance everyone experiences when people move unnecessarily slowly or fail to understand what appears a very simple matter. The difference between the normal person and the patient is that normal people can control their anger, whereas the manic patient may be unable to do so. To help the patient, the nurse should find out what has aroused his anger and avoid irritating him.

DISPLACED ANGER

The anger of an individual patient may not be directed against nurses. It may be aimed at his wife or mother and may arise whenever anyone unconsciously reminds him of the hated person. The nurse may represent a 'mother figure' to the patient, whose hate and aggression are then vented on the nurse. It helps a great deal to remember that in these cases the nurse 'stands for' someone else. If she learns not to take the patient's aggressions any more personally than his affection, she can usually deal with the situation sufficiently calmly and quickly to pacify him. Frequent communication between all those dealing with the patient is necessary in order to understand his attitude and so to be able to modify it.

DELUDED PATIENTS

Some patients are angry about delusional frustrations. If the patient thinks he is being poisoned, he very understandably wishes to protect himself. If he feels threatened he may defend himself. It may not always be possible to predict impulsive behaviour if it arises from a delusional system or if it occurs in response to the command of voices. But though it may not always be possible to predict when a patient will become angry, if the nurse knows him well it may be evident to her that impulsive behaviour may occur. In order to help a patient who suffers from delusions the nurse must know about them and allow the patient to tell his story without contradicting or ridiculing him. If she shows interest and tries to understand how things must appear from the patient's point of view, the patient's behaviour assumes a meaning. When one realizes that he acts as if his delusions were true it is easier to help him.

A patient who feels that people are against him becomes easily angered, suspicious and tense. While the nurse tries to convey to him that she is on his side, and will protect him from any enemies he may believe he has, she may be able to pacify him. If she becomes involved in his delusional system, if he feels that she, too, is in league against him, she is no longer in a good position to help. But at least she knows when this is happening and can be prepared if and when an attack is made.

FACTORS INFLUENCING OUTBREAKS

In any ward in which potentially aggressive patients are nursed, there are occasional outbursts of violent or destructive behaviour. The better the general nursing and management, the fewer these outbursts. When they do occur, they must be dealt with quickly and effectively. When it is all over, nurses should try to find the reason for the disturbance, try to reconstruct the situation in order to see if better observation might have allowed them to predict and so prevent it. The nurses should try to be quite frank in their discussion of the causes of the outburst and should seriously examine their own actions in order to discover to what extent they may have themselves unwittingly provoked it. It is easier to point out to each other where each has gone wrong than to realize personal attitudes. Other people's evaluation of the part each has played should be accepted. This should be done, not in any spirit of criticism, but in an attempt to coordinate the approach to the patient and to prevent recurrence of the incident.

It has been shown that outbursts of violence happen most frequently when the staff are not in agreement about the best approach to the patient or when they do not get on with each other. Possibly their own anxiety and tensions are transmitted to the patient, and he, being less completely in control of his emotions, shows his anxiety in aggressive behaviour.

The really constructive work in a ward of disturbed patients is done when the patients are quiet, for it is at those times that there is an opportunity of building up therapeutic relationships with them. It is at moments of relative calm only that it is possible for the nurse to convince the patient of her interest and ability to help and support him. He can be guided to canalize his energies into acceptable channels. Energetic games and occupations, for instance, can be provided if the patient is physically strong enough to enjoy them.

If the patient is helped to sleep better he may be more relaxed and later more able to tolerate frustrations. On the whole, the atmosphere of the ward depends on the presence of sufficient numbers of efficient, self-confident, calm nurses who convince the patient that they are his friends.

DEALING WITH VIOLENT BEHAVIOUR

However calm and competent, however understanding and tactful nurses may be, they may still at times encounter aggressive and violent behaviour. In order to be able to help the patient, the nurse must know how to deal with any combination of circumstances which may arise. In dealing with the patient she must act in such a way that:

(a) the patient does not suffer physical injury;
(b) the patient does not become exhausted;
(c) other patients are not excessively disturbed by the incident;
(d) other patients are not injured;
(e) the nurses involved are not hurt;

(*f*) property is preserved as far as possible;

(*g*) the patient calms down again quickly after the disturbance.

This last point should be kept in mind throughout the incident. When the disturbance has subsided, the patient feels guilty and frightened, and nurses must do all they can by their attitude to show him that they bear him no ill-feeling. They must convince him that they do not judge his behaviour as being 'bad' or 'wrong'. Their duty is effectively to prevent him from doing harm to himself or others but, having ensured this, they continue to show their liking of the patient and their interest in him, and make efforts to understand him. It must be made as easy as possible for him to calm down without feeling that he has 'lost face' in any way.

Everyone knows from experience how difficult it is to 'climb down' after a quarrel or argument and to take back what has been said. Pride forbids being the first to make a peace offering and so arguments and hostilities are perpetuated, because both parties consider it humiliating to cease. When dealing with a sick person, it would be quite unreasonable, therefore, to expect him to take the initiative in making peace. Nurses lose nothing by offering every conceivable opening to the patient to return to peaceful behaviour.

Weapons Used by Violent Patients

The aims in dealing with violent, excited patients have been listed in the order of importance. But it is useful to deal with them also in reverse order. For many reasons nurses should ensure that property is not excessively destroyed. First, an outburst of destructive behaviour leaves the patient more frightened at the effects he has produced. Second, once furniture and glass is broken, the patient is able to arm himself with dangerous weapons, and inflict injuries upon himself, on other patients and on staff. It is then more difficult later to treat the incident as if it were unimportant. It is therefore sometimes thought advisable that the ward should be suitably equipped for patients who may become violent. Single rooms may be used to isolate a patient if necessary. In these rooms windows should be unbreakable, or shutters could be available to protect the windows and glass panes on doors. The side-room doors should open out-wards so that the patient cannot barricade himself in and should be wide enough to allow furniture to be removed quickly. Some hospitals prefer rooms which have padded floors and walls to protect the patient from injury if he bangs his head or falls. Furniture in the ward should not be easily broken. It may be wise to remove orna-ments which could be thrown or broken, nothing should be left lying about which could become dangerous. Brooms left behind doors, pokers and unnecessary occu-pational tools are all potentially dangerous weapons. In spite of reducing the amount of furniture and the number of ornaments, the ward can be made to look pleasant and comfortable, for example, by using soft furnishings, embroidered cushions and covers and having pictures fixed to the wall.

Handling the Violent Patient

Injury to staff can be prevented only by the most careful team-work. Adequate numbers of nurses are essential, but numbers alone are not enough. Each nurse must know that she can rely with a hundred per cent certainty on the help of the others. She must be able to call for help and obtain it without delay. Each nurse must be prepared to go to the aid of others with the utmost speed.

No nurse should ever attempt to enter single-handed into a struggle with a patient. It is much safer always to leave the patient alone for a moment while getting help. If he should succeed in injuring the nurse, she might then be unable to obtain help. Whenever force is resorted to, there is danger of injury to the patient. The nurse should ensure that she has a witness whenever there is any possibility of her being likely to cause injury or bruising to a patient. The latter may attribute bruises to a nurse when she has not in fact caused them. The hospital is obliged to investigate any complaint against a nurse made by the patient or his relatives, and, even if she has acted with the utmost restraint, she may find it difficult to prove her case without a witness. It is obvious that every injury sustained by a patient or nurse in the course of a struggle should be reported at once and that a written statement should be made by all nurses concerned in the matter.

In order to protect other patients, it is necessary to know which patients do not get on well with each other and, if possible, to separate them before friction arises. The nurse may be able to sense tension in a group of patients and by tactful intervention may prevent major upsets.

Isolation of Violent Patient

Occasionally, but with good nursing only in the rarest circumstances, it may be necessary to lock the door of the patient's room for a while until some better method of dealing with a particular situation can be found.

If the nurse, in an emergency, has locked the door of a patient's room on her own initiative, she must immediately send for the doctor. Some people consider that to lock a patient in is never justified. Others feel that in the defence of other patients it may occasionally be necessary.

The disturbed patient himself very rarely benefits by this in any way. On the contrary, he is likely to become extremely resentful, and this can only increase his aggression, not diminish it. The nurse's attitude can convey to the patient that her action is not meant to be punitive, that it is an emergency measure carried out with regret but with no ill feeling, and that it will be discontinued at the earliest possible moment.

The patient may feel profoundly humiliated by the experience of being locked in and may find it very difficult later to establish any satisfactory relationship with the nurses responsible for this. On the other hand, he may be grateful that he was prevented from causing bodily harm to others and may not harbour resentment against the nurses. Occasionally a patient asks to be locked in his room when he is aware that he is losing control over his actions. He may feel safe in a small, protected room, or he may consider that he is receiving just punishment if he is locked in and then be able to feel less guilty about his actions.

Manual Restraint

In order to prevent the patient from injuring himself, it may be necessary to resort to manual restraint. This is as unpleasant for nurses as for patients and the patient should be aware that the former are reluctant to impose it. If there were the slightest suggestion that nurses enjoyed using force, their position would become quite intolerable. When it is necessary to use restraint, several nurses should be available and act in a co-ordinated effort. They should approach the patient simultaneously, if possible from two sides, and should quickly put him on the bed in the position which will make it easiest to hold him without causing him any discomfort. No more force must be used than is absolutely necessary to keep his movements under control. Nurses should decide beforehand how to approach the patient, so that each knows exactly what to do. It would be folly to take hold of one arm only, because the patient would then hit out with the other. Both arms should be taken at the same time. Movements are best controlled if the large joints are held, i.e. shoulder and hips, rather than wrists or elbows. In order to avoid bruising, a blanket should always be between the nurse's hand and the patient's skin. As soon as possible, the nurses should relax their grip, though they should remain in position to strengthen it if necessary. The fact that they relax almost at once may help to prove their peaceful intentions to the patient. Usually, when there are enough nurses, the patient quickly gives up the struggle. The nurses' attitude should make this easy and as little humiliating as possible. Immediately he has become calmer the difficult task of building up his shattered self-esteem should begin.

CHAPTER 17

Nursing Epileptic Patients

EPILEPSY is a condition in which episodic transient periods of disturbed behaviour or consciousness accompany abnormal electric discharges of the brain. Manifestations of epilepsy vary according to the site and cause of the brain's abnormal functioning. The two commonest forms of epileptic attacks are known as major and minor epilepsy.

MAJOR EPILEPSY

Major epilepsy, or *grand mal*, is characterized by definite stages, beginning with the aura or warning, which is peculiar to each patient and heralds the onset of an attack. The fit is divided into three stages, beginning with the tonic stage in which the patient falls to the ground unconscious and with all his muscles, including the respiratory muscles, in spasm. This stage lasts about thirty seconds and is succeeded by the clonic stage when there are regular jerky movements of the limbs in which the tongue may be bitten by the contractions of the jaw. Incontinence of urine and occasionally of faeces may occur. This stage usually lasts from one to two minutes. The final stage is that of coma, which often passes into sleep lasting for several hours. After an attack the patient's mental state may be one of confusion and he may be violent and aggressive without having any realization of his actions. This is known as 'post-epileptic automatism'.

Minor Epilepsy

Minor epilepsy, or *petit mal*, is characterized by momentary breaks in consciousness without convulsive attacks. The patient ceases any activity in which he is engaged, stares vacantly and may sometimes fall to the ground.

Epileptic Mental Patients

Most people suffering from epilepsy are able to lead a normal life, but a few are admitted to psychiatric hospitals, often for reasons not directly related to their epilepsy. Typical epileptic seizures as described above are rarely observed. Accurate description of each individual patient's seizures is a valuable help in diagnosis and treatment of the condition.

It is often suggested that the nursing care of epileptic patients differs in some respects from that of other psychiatric patients. This is true in so far as observation of fits and the care of the patients during and after fits are concerned. Apart from fits, however, epileptic patients probably have no more symptoms or characteristics in common than other mentally ill patients. In order to give epileptic patients all the care they require it is necessary to know why each patient was admitted to a psychiatric hospital.

Some patients are in psychiatric hospitals because they suffer from some such mental disorder as schizophrenia or depression as well as epilepsy. The nursing care of these is determined by the nature of the mental disorder, although the occurrence of fits creates additional problems. Patients in whom epileptic fits may be due to birth injury may also, for the same reason, suffer from mental subnormality or from an organic psychosis. Both the epilepsy and the mental illness require appropriate treatment. Some epileptic patients have mental disorders which are in some way caused by their epilepsy or related directly to it.

Confusion States

Some patients, before or after fits, undergo periods of confusion when they require skilled supervision lest they come to harm. These periods vary in length and frequency and between them some patients are able to be discharged from hospital. The intervals may always be of the same duration and the patient may be able to arrange to come into hospital when he himself realizes the need. During confused periods he may have difficulty in recognizing familiar people or objects, or may become noisy and destructive. He may be unable to attend to his own toilet or elimination and become incontinent. He may become ill from undernourishment, exposure, injury to the skin and lowered resistance to infection. The patient's physical health requires attention, and, provided he can be nursed successfully during the period of disordered consciousness, he may be able to continue his usual occupation when the confused phase is over.

Some patients' confusion is obvious. Others, however, behave in a manner which gives the impression that they are fully orientated and quite conscious. Later it becomes clear that the patient has complete amnesia for periods during which his consciousness seemed to be complete. The patient's actions are carried out automatically and he cannot later be held responsible for them. Occasionally during these periods he may injure himself or others and he needs protection from the consequence of his actions during these phases.

Emotional States

Some epileptic patients, at the time of fits, or even at other times, find it increasingly difficult to control any emotional reactions which may perhaps unwittingly be aroused by people in the environment. The patient may be irritable, experience hate or anger and, not being able to keep himself under control, may become violent, abusive and dangerous. Moreover, if he feels that he is losing control, he may become extremely frightened. Tension mounts until it becomes intolerable, and an uncontrollable outburst of violence occurs. Nobody enjoys violence, least of all the patient, who afterwards feels guilty and ashamed. He hates himself and hates others for causing him to lose control over himself. Such a patient requires someone who understands him and so can prevent an outburst before it reaches a peak. In a mental hospital this is quite possible. When the nurse knows the patient really well she can usually detect when he is becoming more irritable and tense, and can persuade him to relax. He can be left undisturbed by other patients and the nurse can foster a quiet atmosphere by postponing making any demands on him and refraining from any comment which might upset his control. Sedation well before the storm breaks may be used, or any method of reducing tension known to have been effective on past occasions. The most important of these methods is for the nurse to remain calm, not to show anger or hostility and not to become frightened. This is only possible if she knows the patient well, realizes that he is ill, and treats his aggression as a symptom of his illness. Outside psychiatric hospitals it is not always possible for calmness to reign in the face of a patient's aggressive behaviour. The patient and his environment react on each other until real danger exists which in hospital can be prevented.

Some epileptic patients, who have been taking anti-convulsant drugs for some time, begin to show mental symptoms, often resembling those of mania, or they may occasionally display the features of confusional illness or of dementia. It is sometimes necessary to withdraw the drugs in order to establish to what extent symptoms are due to drug intoxication, and also to what extent drugs are really necessary to keep the fits under control. During this period the patient requires continuous observation and very careful nursing.

Behaviour Disorders

By far the greatest number of epileptic patients are in psychiatric hospitals because of behaviour disturbances. Over a period of time the patient's behaviour may have become so difficult that it is impossible for him to remain in the community. It is possible, though no conclusive evidence exists, that some forms of epileptic illnesses lead to a progressive deterioration in behaviour and to a characteristic kind of personality disorder.

Patients suffering from 'temporal lobe epilepsy' sometimes show a characteristic form of disorder which often responds well to surgical removal of the epileptic focus in the temporal lobe. Restlessness, irritability, slow circumstantial speech and episodic outbursts of aggressive behaviour are common.

Often, however, behaviour disorder is not the result of epileptic illness, but a reaction to the way in which the patient is treated by society. Whatever the cause, the nurse will find it much easier to remedy the patient's behaviour if she assumes that it is the result of environmental influences. It used to be believed that epileptic patients were people whose personality showed antisocial characteristics. If, before she ever approaches the patient, the nurse believes that epileptics are hypocrites, schemers, liars and generally untrustworthy people, her attitude will show diffidence and suspicion of their every action, which may then result in bringing out in them the very characteristics she has expected. If, however, she assumes that the patients are kindly disposed, pleasant and likeable people, her approach to them will be much more natural, spontaneous and friendly, and they may respond by differing very little from other groups of patients.

It is very easy, if one is suspicious of people, to create a situation which is self-verifying. The way in which one approaches a person of whom one is suspicious creates in that person hostility and aggression he had not previously felt. The moment these feelings emerge they serve to confirm that the suspicions were justified.

It is possible that in the past nurses created among epileptic patients the behaviour and personality traits of which they were afraid.

Epileptic Children

Nurses who do meet an epileptic patient who is sly, treacherous, deceitful and untrustworthy should try to think of the kind of social life people suffering from epilepsy are liable to lead. From the moment fits have occurred, be it in childhood or later, the patient is prevented from leading a normal life. Fits are very terrifying to witness. Undoubtedly the child's parents are most upset when they first discover that he has had a fit. They communicate their anxiety to the child, who is disturbed by the sudden inexplicable attacks and feels that something is happening over which he has no control. Once the diagnosis of epilepsy is made, the parents are in a greater dilemma than ever. They are worried, feel guilty and responsible and seek in the child's antenatal history, or in heredity, an explanation for the illness. They become over-solicitous, restrictive and at the same time over-indulgent. They may wish to protect the child from injury by keeping careful watch, but at the same time they prevent normal activity in sports and games, and never let the child out of their sight. They may feel frightened, possibly even repelled by the fits, and will probably be a little resentful about the difficulties created in their lives by the fact that an epileptic child must be cared for. It is a great strain to bring up an epileptic child, especially where there are several children in the family and, however devoted the parents, the child must sometimes realize how much inconvenience he causes.

School represents a problem. If the child has frequent fits, ordinary schools will not admit him. Even if they did, the child would soon fall behind in his work as a result of repeated absences. If he has minor epileptic fits, the position may even be worse; the fits are often not recognized and the child is thought to be lazy, absent-minded and clumsy, and is subjected to criticism and ridicule. Since he cannot control the fits, he becomes despondent and gives up trying, or may become resentful, angry and aggressive. If an epileptic child goes to an ordinary school he probably feels different, an outsider, an oddity. He may be excluded from many activities and soon realizes that the other children are frightened of or amused by his fits and shun his company on their parents' advice. If the child goes to one of the special boarding schools for epileptic children he benefits educationally, but family life is disrupted and this may give rise to many of the patient's later difficulties.

The Epileptic in Society

As an adult, the epileptic finds life just as difficult. Many jobs are out of the question for him. It would be most unwise for anyone who is liable to have fits to drive a bus or a car, or to choose any occupation which requires climbing ladders or handling dangerous machinery. The number of occupations from which he can choose is limited, but even if he selects one which is well within his powers he may meet with fear and prejudice on the part of his potential employer. If he tells the employer that he has fits he may not be accepted. If he does not tell him, he may be dealt with even less sympathetically when his employer discovers the situation. It is not really surprising that some epileptic patients, because of their experiences, become asocial, if not actually antisocial. Some feel that the world is against them and see no reason why they should consider themselves as being a part of society which has rejected them.

The Epileptic in Hospital

Even in a psychiatric hospital, although the epileptic's plight is understood and appreciated, there are difficulties in deciding on how to treat him. If all epileptic patients are placed in one ward, an entirely arbitrary criterion is used for selection. Patients who have fits may have very little else in common. Some are severely psychotic, some mentally subnormal, some disturbed, others normal most of the time and merely in need of short periods of supervision. It is unlikely that the patients can form a group, or benefit from psychiatric hospital treatment in the way other patients do, if they are in the same ward merely because they have fits. If, on the other hand, the epileptic patient is admitted to any other ward, he again finds himself an outsider, an object of pity and curiosity, not an accepted member of the group. He is again restricted in his activities and barred from certain occupations. In view of all this, it is not surprising that epileptic patients are sometimes difficult people to manage. It is much more surprising that they lose their temper so rarely, and fit in as well as they do, sometimes becoming some of the most efficient and the most reliable members of the ward community.

NURSING EPILEPTIC PATIENTS

The nursing care of the epileptic patient may be considered under two headings:

(1) the general management of the patient within the hospital;

(2) the special care required in view of the occurrence of fits.

(1) The general management should be planned with regard to the patient's mental and physical condition. The patient should share as fully as possible in the life of the community. If his fits are well under control there should be little difficulty in finding suitable work and arranging a full occupational and recreational programme, although it must be remembered that a certain amount of supervision is always necessary and the patient should not be allowed to work in any place where a fit might endanger the lives of others.

(2) So far as fits are concerned, the following nursing aspects should be considered:

    (a) Observation and investigation of fits.
    (b) Prevention of fits.
    (c) Care and management during fits.

These three aspects are closely connected and dependent on each other. Fits are more easily prevented if they have been carefully investigated and described. Management during a fit is similarly dependent on accurate observation.

Observation of Fits

Investigations are carried out in hospital because it is essential to obtain the report of trained observers, and also because certain tests, e.g. electroencephalography and metabolic investigations, may be required in order to establish the diagnosis and to guide treatment.

From relatives it may be impossible to obtain an accurate description of what has actually taken place during fits they have observed. This is due to the following reasons: first, it is impossible for those who are upset and worried to observe accurately, and relatives are invariably upset by the circumstances. Second, it is impossible to remember accurately what has been observed unless observations are at once committed to writing, before any distortion has taken place, and unless it is realized at the time of observation that a report will later be required. Third, it is impossible accurately to remember every detail. Some selection is determined by what the observer considers to be of importance. The popular idea of what is of importance may not always correspond with the actual requirements of the doctor.

The nurse's observation can be more accurate because she acts as the trained observer, who bears these points in mind and systematically sets out to provide what is needed. At first, even the nurse may be upset and excited and the first reports are therefore not always very accurate. They serve a useful purpose if the nurse tries to compare her observations with those of another nurse who has also witnessed the fit and attempts to find out whether her own observations were biased.

After the first experiences, the nurse should be able to remain calm and her observation should improve. The main reason for inaccurate reporting after the first few occasions may be the fact that fits occasionally occur when the nurse is not prepared, and that at times she is taken by surprise. She may feel that she should have been prepared, that she has not been sufficiently vigilant. She may feel guilty because she has failed to observe the onset of the fit or the circumstances which have led up to it. She should not allow her feelings in this case to influence her report, and should resist the temptation of reporting what might have been. She should adhere strictly to facts actually observed. A few fits really well observed are a much better guide to the doctor than a large number of reports which are inaccurate.

As soon as possible after the fit, the nurse must find time to write down her observations. While the fit is actually in progress she should give a verbal running commentary to herself of what is happening. This helps the later writing of the report. Most doctors give the nurse a series of headings under which a report is to be made and the nurse should memorize these in order to have a reply to each question.

As soon as she observes a patient who has a fit, the nurse should note the time, because she should report accurately on the total length of the fit and the length of each stage. Time may seem very long when she is helplessly watching a patient and the period during which the patient is not breathing may seem endless, when in fact it may last only thirty seconds.

The nurse should prepare a summary of the condition of the ward as she finds it and remember what the patient had been doing just prior to the fit. Fits may occur more frequently when a patient is upset. There may be some relation to the intake of food and it is a help if the existence of some recurrent antecedent activity can be established. Some patients, for example, are most likely to have fits when there has been some quarrel or unpleasant scene in the ward. Others regularly have fits during hospital concerts or in the ward when someone plays the piano. Sometimes it is even one particular tune which is associated with the onset of a fit. Any precipitating factors in the environment should be noted as well as the patient's own mood or activity just before the seizure.

If the patient is regularly irritable immediately prior to an attack, this may be an expression of his own awareness of an impending attack. The irregular electric discharge of the brain may occur from the onset of irritability. Noticing this may help in foreseeing an attack and in better management of future seizures. Any warning the patient may have should be noted. He may communicate this in words at the time or later, or he may indicate it by some specific action which always precedes an attack.

Loss of consciousness or disturbance of consciousness should be reported. The nurse should practise making the necessary observations swiftly and in correct order, to establish the level of consciousness and whether the unconscious state is deepening or becoming less deep. She should call the patient's name, noting any utterances which may give evidence of his having heard or observed the nurse. She should report posture or the succession of postures, the movement of the head and eyes, the direction of movement. The direction of the fall should be noted. The exact length of time of each stage of the attack is important. Muscle tone should be observed, whether the tonic or rigid stage is unilateral or bilateral, whether twitching starts simultaneously throughout the whole body, or on which side or which part of the body it appears first. Twitching may start at one particular point and spread from there, and the order in which various parts of the body are affected may be important. Muscle tone at the end of the attack should be noted. The eyes should be observed. The reaction of pupils to light, corneal reflexes and eye movements must be mentioned.

As soon as the attack has ceased, pulse and respiration are recorded, colour is noted. Biting of the tongue and incontinence are reported, knee jerks and Babinski reflexes are tested. (Babinski's sign is an upward movement of the big toe when the sole of the foot is stroked. Normally the toe moves downward.) After the attack it is necessary to note the depth of the sleep which follows, how easy it is to rouse the patient, and the duration of sleep if the patient is left undisturbed. Any complaints made by the patient are reported, e.g. headache or vomiting, so is any evidence of confusion in speech or action. It is very important to establish the length of time during which the patient remains confused because during it he requires supervision and is not responsible for his actions. The patient may appear to be fully conscious, but later questioning may reveal a period of amnesia at a time when confusion was not evident.

Electroencephalography

Observations of the kind described may give an indication of the localization of a brain lesion or of the metabolic disturbance which may cause the fits. The observation of fits may be supplemented by the investigation of the electrical discharge of the brain under a variety of conditions. Electric brain waves have been widely discussed in the popular press, and many patients now arrive in hospital with some vague notion about the tests which are performed. They approach the investigations with preconceived ideas of the purpose of the test. Some patients fear that electricity is being used on the brain, having confused 'E.C.T.' and 'E.E.G.'. The use of abbreviations adds to the mystery of the subject and many patients are terrified of the technique. It is bad for the patient to worry unnecessarily if a few words of reassurance and explanation can allay his fears. Worry may interfere seriously with the result of the test because the patient may be restless when he arrives at the electroencephalography department, or in some instances may even refuse to have the test done. The patient who is struggling and restless may require sedation prior to investigation, and this may be undesirable. Some patients have exaggerated ideas of the efficacy of the E.E.G. test and believe that their most secret thoughts may be revealed. Not unnaturally these patients may be reluctant to have the test done. The nurse can find out how much the patient knows about the test, and should then correct misconceptions. She should seek guidance from the doctor before she assures the patient that the test is completely painless, as some special tests, e.g. overbreathing during E.E.G., sphenoidal E.E.G., or E.E.G.

accompanied by light flicker or Metrazol, can be intensely uncomfortable.

(In sphenoidal E.E.G., electrodes are passed through skin and subcutaneous tissue to reach the base of the skull and enable recordings to be made from the inferior part of the temporal lobe of the brain.)

PREVENTION OF FITS

Accurate descriptions of the fits, together with reports of the electroencephalogram give guidance to the doctor in his prescription of drugs. As the drugs take effect the characteristic features of the fits may change. To assess the efficacy of the drugs prescribed, continued careful reporting of the incidence of fits and a description of them remains important.

Fits are often found to be related to emotional disturbances. Their incidence may be reduced if the patient is well adjusted to his environment, happy in his personal relationships with other patients, doctors and nurses, and if the ward atmosphere is generally congenial to him. A sudden increase in the number of fits may be an indication of the patient's unfavourable reaction to changes in staff or routine, and it may be possible to readjust his environment if this possibility is borne in mind. If the patient's fits are to remain controlled after discharge, it is important that the patient should have the opportunity of testing his adaptation to work and home life while still under the supervision of the hospital.

Diet and fluid intake are sometimes found to be related to fits. If it is found that these occur with fluid retention diuretics may be ordered, or the patient may have his fluids restricted. If fits occur frequently during the night it may be necessary to restrict fluid intake in the evenings. Slight hypoglycaemia may bring on fits. Frequent small meals during the day and a milky drink late in the evening may reduce their incidence. While prevention of fits is not always possible, careful nursing and attention to detail can considerably reduce their number and consequently enable the patient to lead a more normal life.

PRECAUTIONS AGAINST INJURY

During a fit the most important duty of the nurse is to prevent injury. Epileptic patients in hospital are kept under fairly constant observation day and night. Certain obvious dangers are avoided. Fires are guarded so that burns, the most common injuries outside hospital, rarely occur. The patient may sleep on a low bed so that he would not be injured if he fell out, but this is seldom necessary. He has a hard pillow, in order not to suffocate if his face happened to be covered by the pillow during a fit. Meals are supervised in case a fit occurs, and the patient is encouraged to cut up his food into small pieces because he might choke if a fit occurred while large pieces of food were in his mouth. The patient is never alone in the bathroom, since there is some risk of drowning. He should have no opportunity to climb heights. The dangers of traffic are obviated if the patient goes out only when accompanied.

Ward furnishings should be so arranged that the risk of injury during falls is minimized. Low, well-upholstered armchairs and rugs on the floor may help. There should be plenty of loose cushions which can be used especially if the patient falls to the ground. Patients frequently help each other, and should be encouraged to do so, at least to move the patient to a place of safety, or to guide or break his fall. Each patient will feel more secure if he sees that accidents are few and that his fellow patients are cared for and safely attended to during a fit. The patient needs to judge for himself how great the risk of injury is and how far it is advisable to take calculated risks in order to prepare for discharge.

Risk from Drugs

Since most epileptic patients are taking drugs of some kind the nurses who work in these wards should be familiar not only with the method of administration of drugs but particularly with the possible toxic effects of each. Nurses who know that excessive drowsiness may result from phenobarbitone will be more alert to changes in the patient's behaviour, and will report his reluctance to go to occupational classes or to join in social activities. If the patient is having Epanutin she will keep a special watch for spongy gums, and attend more carefully to the patient's oral hygiene. She must bear in mind that the noisy, talkative, excited patient may be suffering from the ill effects of the drug. Some drugs given to epileptic patients cause occasional visual hallucinations. Skin rashes are common, and blood counts may be necessary because certain drugs cause a reduction in the number of white blood cells and this would predispose the patient to infection.

After discharge, sufferers from epilepsy continue to take anticonvulsant drugs, for many years, sometimes for the rest of their life. Knowledge about the drugs is therefore as important to the patient as it is to the nurse. The patient should know the names of the drugs he is taking, the dosage which has been prescribed for him and the importance of taking the drugs regularly. He should understand that regular medication is necessary to maintain the required drug level in the blood. Some patients mistakenly believe that they can take a double or treble dose one day if they forget to take the drugs on other days. The danger and uselessness of this procedure should be made clear to the patient. Though prolonged taking of drugs on medical prescription is not only safe for the patient, but necessary, the same drugs may be dangerous if taken by other people. The patient should be fully aware of his responsibility for the safe keeping of his drugs when he leaves the hospital.

There is danger in the hospital care of epileptic patients that nurses retain full responsibility for too long.

The patient suffering from epilepsy needs to be fully involved in the planning of his life after discharge. He must be prepared for the harsh reality of the difficulties of obtaining suitable employment, the embarrassment of meeting tactless or unhelpful people, the problems of preventing injury. The hospital should offer him every opportunity to learn how to do without its support.

CHAPTER 18

Patients who are Dependent on Drugs or Alcohol

ALCOHOLISM is a disorder which is common in many countries. The extent to which it is recognised as a social or medical problem depends on the prevailing attitude of the community.

It has long been recognised as a medical problem when people who have taken alcohol regularly over a long period of time, come to suffer from brain damage and accompanying mental deterioration or from other bodily damage. Increasingly, psychiatrists and psychiatric nurses are becoming aware, not only of body damage caused by alcohol, but of the difficulties of people whose lives are largely dominated by thoughts about drinking. Such people are addicted to alcohol. How many people are alcohol addicts is not known, but it is generally agreed that the prevalence of alcoholism is quite considerable.

By contrast, drug addiction was, until recently, thought to be uncommon in the United Kingdom. In recent years the incidence of drug addiction appears to have increased and many people express growing concern about this. Discussions about this problem are, however, confused because no clear definition is used for the concept of addiction. Some people, for example, make no distinction between alcohol addicts and heavy drinkers, others believe that a distinction can be drawn.

Some people make no distinction between 'habituation' to drugs and drug 'addiction'. Others distinguish between habituation, i.e. the need for increasing dosage of drugs to achieve the same effect, and addiction, i.e. the craving for the drug and the inability to do without it.

In order to remove some of the difficulty of definition and in order to make possible international comparison of the incidence of the disorder and of the effectiveness of treatment, the World Health Organization recommended in 1964 in a technical report (No. 287) that the word 'addiction' should be replaced by the term 'drug dependence'. This term describes much better than the word 'addiction' the central preoccupation of the patients who are totally dependent on a regular supply of their drug of addiction, be it alcohol or any other drug. The use of the term 'dependence' encourages one to concentrate on the patients' needs rather than on the pharmacological characteristics of the drug or on legal definition.

Patients suffering from dependence on drugs or alcohol have certain problems in common:

(1) By the time dependence is established the patients are able to take much more of the drug without showing any ill-effects, than would be possible for other people. Patients dependent on alcohol, for example, can sometimes drink two bottles of whisky without showing signs of being drunk. Patients dependent on sedatives take doses so large that others would be made unconscious. Patients dependent on heroin need ever larger doses to give them the sensation which they hope for. This phenomenon is known as *tolerance*. The ability to acquire tolerance to drugs such as morphine and heroin was always known and some of them were classified by the Dangerous Drugs Acts as drugs of addiction. No drugs, however, are entirely safe—tolerance to dexedrine, methedrine, aspirin, barbiturates and alcohol is quite as common

as tolerance to the drugs named in the Dangerous Drugs Acts.

(2) Patients who are dependent on drugs or alcohol usually experience intense *craving* when the next dose is not immediately available. A patient suffering from the later stages of alcoholism wakes up in the morning feeling shaky, restless and nauseated. He is unable to start the business of the day until he has had a drink. Periodically throughout the day this feeling comes over him again. When the addiction has progressed farther, to obtain his drink quickly he keeps a secret stock of drink in his office and from time to time, all by himself, he takes a drink. As soon as he has had a drink the shaky, trembling sensation leaves him. Because he knows he can make himself feel better by drinking, the patient's social life tends to be dominated by his need to obtain a drink. He arrives at parties early, to have one drink before the others start, he drops in at a pub on his way home from work. Many patients who suffer from alcoholism are never able to be entirely without alcohol in their circulation. For some alcoholics, known as *bout drinkers*, the craving is only intermittent. They are able to go for weeks or months without a drink, but when a drinking bout starts the craving is paramount.

Craving for other drugs is more difficult to satisfy than craving for alcohol. Unless the drugs are prescribed by a doctor at a special clinic, the patient finds he can obtain his supply only through illegal activities. In order to ensure a supply he must then make contacts with the people who are able to get access to such supplies; consequently he quickly finds himself at the mercy of unscrupulous people who can ask for ever-increasing amounts of money for the drugs, or blackmail the drug dependent patient into participating in criminal activities. What may have started as an experiment to see if some 'kicks' could be obtained, may end in a life of crime, revolving round the problem of obtaining supplies of drugs.

Many people believe that the dangers involved in participating in illegal trafficking of drugs are greater than the dangers of drug taking themselves. They would wish to see drugs, particularly 'soft' drugs such as hashish ('pot'), more freely available, as is the case with alcohol, so that people dependent on drugs need not resort to crime to obtain them. There is, however, a considerable danger that, in a free market for drugs, drug dependence might become as common as alcohol dependence. It is one of the most worrying aspects of the problem of drug taking that many young people appear to start with the relatively harmless drugs which are more easily obtainable, e.g., methedrine, dexedrine and the smoking of hashish, and find themselves pushed by the people whose company they keep into dependence on hard drugs, like heroin.

(3) The most serious symptoms which may arise occur when the patient is no longer able to obtain the drug on which he depends. These symptoms are referred to as the *withdrawal state*. The shakes and tremors described above constitute withdrawal symptoms. Withdrawal symptoms are very similar in patients suffering from alcoholism and from drug dependence. Restlessness, agitation, terrifying hallucinations are among the most prominent symptoms. When the delirium is gross, the patient may be disorientated; he may be quite unable to remember where he is and how he got there. He may mistake people in the hospital for relatives or friends, and may restlessly carry out activities which may be quite exhausting and damaging in view of his poor physical health. Epileptiform fits may occur.

In patients suffering from alcoholism these withdrawal symptoms are referred to as delirium tremens.

When a patient who is a habitual drinker is admitted to a general hospital after an accident or for an operation delirium tremens occurs because the withdrawal of alcohol is sudden. It is a particularly dangerous condition when it occurs as a complication to an already serious surgical condition, and must be quickly brought under control by the administration of tranquillizing drugs, e.g., Largactil mg. 100 t.d.s. For patients commencing treatment for alcoholism or for drug dependence, the withdrawal symptoms are equally severe and sometimes prove to be so insufferable that the patient prefers to discontinue treatment. Withdrawal symptoms can be kept under control by the use of large doses of tranquillizers, but very careful nursing attention is required to deal with the restlessness and confusion and to guard against injury. Dehydration and intercurrent infections are possible complications of withdrawal symptoms.

Because alcohol is readily available, while the sale of other drugs of addiction is legally restricted, it is easier to become addicted to alcohol than to other drugs, and easier to reach an advanced stage of dependence before the need for medical aid is recognised. Until fairly recently it was not as difficult as is generally believed, however, to obtain doctors' prescriptions for habit-forming drugs in large enough quantities to be able to sell off some of the surplus, and perhaps this is the reason why the incidence of drug addiction has increased considerably in the last few years.

In 1965 a committee, under the chairmanship of Lord Brain, recommended that the right of prescribing certain specified drugs should be limited to a number of doctors working in special clinics. These clinics came into being in April 1968 and all addicts will now be officially registered. This will make it much easier to estimate the magnitude of the problem, to limit the availability of 'hard' drugs, and to carry out research into the effectiveness of treatment.

Research is also necessary to find out how serious is the danger of dependence on 'hard' drugs for those who have taken 'soft' drugs such as cannabis. Many people dependent on heroin are known to have started with 'soft' drugs, but it is not known how many people experiment with cannabis, hashish or L.S.D. without coming to any harm, and without proceeding to 'hard' drugs. It would appear that among students for example, experimentation with soft drugs is fairly common. Young people often have the desire to extend their experience. The effects of some drugs such as L.S.D. on perception and feeling have been extensively described. To many people these experiences are pleasurable and even awe inspiring. To some they are a welcome escape from the tedium of everyday life, to others they represent a more positive almost mystical, awareness of a reality worth exploring for its own sake.

There appear to be many people who grow tired of the experience and give up drugs without any difficulty. Others may not find it so easy and may need help. For this purpose it is necessary that they should feel free to discuss their problems and should know where to turn for help.

While the taking of all drugs is regarded as blameworthy, wicked or degenerate, and while all of it is illegal, it is difficult for drugtakers to disclose their need for help early enough. There is no means of spotting those who take drugs in the early stages. The need for help must be made known by the drugtaker himself or by his friends.

Treatment and Nursing Care

Treatment of patients suffering from drug dependence can rarely be successfully undertaken unless the patient wishes to be helped. Many patients agree to see a psychiatrist in order to satisfy their employer or their spouse, or they enter hospital under pressure from friends or from a magistrate. Such patients are unlikely to persevere with treatment when the withdrawal symptoms become troublesome or when they experience craving for the drug. When the patient himself has come to the conclusion that he must seek help, such help is more likely to be effective. Unfortunately, many people who are dependent on drugs require the sensations of euphoria, heightened confidence in themselves, emotional upsurge and enlarged perception which the drugs bring about. They may also value their place in the circle of friends into whose company their drug dependence brings them, and they are not able to make a change. It used to be said by 'Alcoholics Anonymous' that it is only when a patient reaches rock-bottom, when he is financially ruined, when his family have left him or when his physical health is seriously impaired, that he genuinely sees the need for treatment. Even then and with the best will in the world, some patients find it impossible to persevere with treatment and succumb time and time again to the temptation of another dose.

Patients suffering from drug addiction and those suffering from alcoholism are increasingly referred to psychiatric clinics for treatment. Often regular attendance at outpatients' clinics gives them the necessary support, especially when an interested social worker can assist in solving the financial and social difficulties into which their addiction has led them. Group psychotherapy is sometimes available to patients attending outpatients' clinics.

Many patients are, however, admitted as inpatients, some into psychiatric admission wards where they are treated alongside patients with other psychological problems, some into special units for the treatment of their addiction.

In special units patients find support from other patients. They can help each other to explore their difficulties and can develop a common culture within the unit. They can benefit from the feeling of being understood and they can examine their reactions and attitudes in the presence of others like themselves. Staff in such units work there because they have special interest in patients suffering from addiction and are more able than others to understand the patients' difficulties.

Patients who are in wards with other in-patients often feel that they are misunderstood by staff and patients alike. Where the demands made by other psychiatric patients have priority the nurses may find patients suffering from drug dependence a nuisance. The craving for the drug and the patient's occasional failure to remain abstinent may be interpreted as non-cooperation.

The advantage of being treated in a ward alongside other psychiatric patients may lie in preventing isolation from society as a whole. It may also be easier to control the supply of drugs from outside the hospital. Where a number of patients suffering from drug dependence are treated together it is easy to find some means of having supplies brought in without the knowledge of the staff. Some patients in fact may leave hospital having been put in touch with better sources of supply than had been available before admission.

The aim of group therapy, however, should be to bring such problems into the open for discussion: this is much less likely to happen in a ward with patients suffering from other psychiatric disorders.

In the nursing care of patients suffering from drug dependence, all the skills described in earlier chapters are required.

(1) The first stage of treatment is concerned with the withdrawal of drugs or with 'drying out' from

alcohol. Much of the nurses' contribution consists of physical care. Drugs have to be administered, and the patient's nutrition needs attention—often the patient is unwilling to take adequate food or fluid because he feels so sick and is so restless. Vitamin deficiency is one of the complications which result from prolonged existence on inadequate diet on which many patients relied prior to admission.

(2) The intense amount of physical nursing care required by the patient during this phase facilitates the creation of an interpersonal relationship between nurse and patient which may be helpful. Patients who have been using drugs or alcohol for a long time often feel that no one trusts them and that they can trust no one. It is helpful to the patient to find a nurse who really listens to him and who is willing to try and understand his side of the story. Some patients have serious personality difficulties and the opportunity to talk about these to a sympathetic nurse may be very valuable. The patient may benefit, not so much from the reply which the nurse offers, as from her continued accepting response even when she learns of the priority he gave to drinking, his sexual problems or his neglect of his family. Many patients feel intensely remorseful and need the opportunity to sort out their feelings by talking about them. The nurse who listens may make it easier for him to do this. It should be remembered that suicide is common in patients who suffer from drug dependence. Evidence of a suicidal impulse may be detected by the nurse who knows how to listen.

(3) The most important aspect of treatment may be the creation in the ward of a new environment in which the patient can make friends and find other satisfactions. To give up drinking or drugs may mean cutting oneself off from the people with whom one previously had social intercourse. The nurse's contri-

bution to the patient's treatment may lie chiefly in helping to create the ward atmosphere in which the patient can feel free from tensions. Interest in work and in hobbies can be encouraged: a new purposive way of living can be established. Ward meetings can be used to help the patient discover his social skills. Group psychotherapy helps him to see his specific personality problems and share these with his fellow sufferers.

Many patients who suffer from drug dependence feel that they are outcasts from society. They create for themselves a defence against 'them', i.e. all the people who are against them and who don't understand. In the right kind of therapeutic milieu this attitude can be avoided or overcome.

It is often difficult to achieve the amount of understanding which the patient needs in order to regain his self respect. Often when the patient speaks of the people who dislike him and who are against him, there is more than a grain of truth in his complaint. The patient's behaviour prior to admission may have strained relationships to near breaking point. His overriding need for his drug or for alcohol while in hospital may result in behaviour which appears to the nurses and to other patients as unreliable and deceitful. It is part of the characteristic pattern of the disorder that these difficulties arise, and part of the treatment that one needs to persevere in spite of setbacks and disappointments.

When the patients leave hospital they may still be faced with formidable problems. Membership of Alcoholics Anonymous, or of similar lay groups of drug addicts, may help them to obtain the necessary support. It is often possible to put the patient in touch with such organizations while he is still in hospital.

There may be many social problems which contributed

to the patient becoming dependent. The patient's job may, for example, be such that alcohol cannot be avoided, or the patient's wife may be a competent, managing person, who really feels happier when her husband is ill than when he copes well with his affairs.

It may be useful to extend treatment to other members of the patient's family. During the patient's stay in hospital group meetings in which members of the family participate may help everyone to understand mutual problems more clearly and to see how far complaints made about each other are valid and realistic. Fellow patients may help to put the problems of the spouse. The patient's relatives may come to accept drug dependence as an illness and may become more able to give sympathy and understanding in spite of all their trials and tribulations.

The continued support and interest from the treatment team may be necessary if the patient is to continue a life of abstinence after leaving hospital.

This support may be offered by the social worker who may continue to visit the patient. It may be given by the doctor in the form of supportive psychotherapy. Some hospitals encourage patients to continue attendance at group psychotherapy sessions for some time after discharge.

It may be that the nurse who has gained the patient's and the relatives' confidence during his stay in hospital is the person to whom the patient can turn again later for support.

Books for Further Reading

General Introduction to Psychiatry and to Psychiatric Nursing

B. R. Ackner (Ed.). (1961) *Handbook for Psychiatric Nurses.* R.M.P.A. and Baillière, Tindall and Cassell, London.

M. M. Glatt and others. (1967) *The Drug Scene in Great Britain.* Arnold, London.

N. Kessel and H. Walton. (1965) *Alcoholism.* Penguin Books, Harmondsworth.

R. R. Mezer and S. Stanner. (1963) *Elements of Psychiatry for Nurses.* Heinemann, London.

W. L. Linford Rees. (1967) *A Short Textbook of Psychiatry.* English Universities Press, London.

D. Stafford-Clark. (1964) *Psychiatry Today.* 2nd ed. Penguin books, Harmondsworth.

M. Valentine. (1965) *Introduction to Psychiatry.* 3rd ed. Livingstone, Edinburgh.

Biographies and Experiences of Mentally Ill Patients

Clifford W. Beers. (1948) *The Mind that Found Itself.* Doubleday, New York.

J. Custance. (1951) *Wisdom, Madness and Folly.* Gollancz, London.

J. Evans. (1954) *Three Men.* Gollancz, London.

P. Hackett. (1953) *The Cardboard Giants.* Gollancz, London.

J. H. Ogdon. (1947) *Kingdom of the Lost.* John Lane, London.

C. M. Wallace. (1965) *Portrait of a Schizophrenic Nurse.* Hammond, London.

PART II

SPECIAL FORMS OF
TREATMENT

CHAPTER 19

Physical Treatment

PHYSICAL treatment in psychiatry serves a variety of purposes. Its value, in some respects, is undisputed. In other respects psychiatrists differ in the importance they attach to physical treatment.

In Chapter 3 it was pointed out that there are three fundamentally different approaches to psychiatric treatment. The importance attached to physical, social and psychological factors in the causation of mental disorder determines the attitude to physical treatment.

There can be no doubt that historically, physical treatment has played an important part in the changing pattern of psychiatric care.

Until a few years ago patients admitted to psychiatric hospitals received no other care than the general nursing which the staff were able to give. With careful attention to the patient's physical health and general custodial care, hospital life offered the best opportunity for patients to recover spontaneously; the sympathy and kindness of the staff undoubtedly helped in speeding this process. When patients were occupied, improvement and recovery were found to be rapid and frequent and a substantial number of patients were discharged within a few years. Many more might have been discharged if contact with the family had not been lost.

Although the outlook was by no means hopeless it was generally thought to be so. Patients believed that they would never be discharged, once they had been admitted to a psychiatric hospital. Relatives feared that the prospects were hopeless, and were at first reluctant to do anything which could be instrumental in 'putting the patient away', with the result that treatment was delayed until the patient's illness was at an advanced stage when the prognosis was less good than it might have been. The idea that the prospects were hopeless was also prevalent among those who worked in psychiatric hospitals and even more so among those who declined, because of this, to work in such institutions.

With the advent of physical treatments the outlook changed abruptly and hope was introduced into the atmosphere of the hospital. Although some early claims for the various treatments were exaggerated, the introduction of each new treatment gave a new impetus to research. Since many of the physical treatments were potentially dangerous it was essential to have well-trained nursing staff and the introduction of such well-trained staff contributed considerably to the raised morale of the hospitals. Most important of all, the attitude of patients and relatives changed. Each felt that in physical treatment lay the great hope for dramatic cure, and patients began to clamour for 'treatment', any treatment, as long as 'something was being done'.

The stage has now been reached when the value of physical treatment is recognized by the public, but doctors and nurses also recognize its limitations. Patients and their relatives continue to build up hopes in relation to physical treatment only, and are often quite incapable of realizing that anything is being done for the patient if this type of therapy is withheld. Over and over again patients who are receiving intensive psychotherapy ask 'When am I going to have treatment?' and it is even common for nurses to ask similar questions about patients who are being treated by psychological and environmental methods.

While it may be very difficult for the patient to realize

the value of occupational therapy or the influence of social therapy, it is most essential that the nurse should be fully aware of the fact that physical treatment is not usually 'the' treatment, it is only one small part of the whole, although the relative importance of this and all other therapeutic measures employed varies with each individual patient.

There are psychiatrists who believe that physical treatment should be administered to most patients for the psychological benefit they derive from it. In some European countries, for example, hydrotherapy is extensively used for this purpose. New psychiatric hospitals are being built in which a physiotherapy department constitutes a major section. A variety of tub baths, showers, packs, steam and sauna baths are available and massage is an important part of treatment.

In the United Kingdom this form of physical treatment has never been much in vogue. However, the psychological effect of other forms of physical treatment, for example, insulin therapy or drug therapy, is much emphasized.

At the present time physical treatment in psychiatry is used for one of three reasons:

(a) There are many psychiatrically ill patients whose physical health is not good and who benefit from physical treatment, particularly if such treatment is aimed at providing rest and improving nutrition.

(b) In some mental disorders, certain forms of physical treatment have been found to work though little is known of their specific effect. Electroconvulsive therapy, for example, is known to relieve depression. Prefontal leucotomy is known to lead to considerable improvement in some patients. Empirical use of physical treatments is justified to relieve suffering pending better understanding of their mode of action.

(c) Some forms of physical treatment are based on

research findings. Drugs, for example, are used in psychiatry in an increasingly scientific manner.

In the chapters which follow, each of these three aspects will be discussed. Physical treatment no longer widely used in this country will not be described in detail. Should, at any time, detailed knowledge of the administration of such treatment be necessary, a number of books can be consulted, a list of which can be found at the end of each chapter.

CHAPTER 20

Continuous Narcosis Therapy, Modified Insulin Therapy and Prolonged Baths

FOR patients whose physical condition is poor, one or other of the treatments described in this chapter may be used. These treatments prevent over-activity, arrest loss of weight and help the patient to regain strength.

CONTINUOUS NARCOSIS THERAPY

Because the treatment is given for reasons which can be easily explained to the patient and easily understood both by him and his relatives, there need be no undue apprehension. It is usually wisest to avoid the use of the term 'narcosis' and use the expression 'sleep treatment', telling the patient that it will give him increased rest and care, and that he will soon improve.

Many patients feel that 'rest' is what they really require and, although in many mental disorders this is not the case, it is true of patients whose energy output is excessive e.g. those who are anxious and who therefore readily appreciate the need for rest and welcome relief from insomnia. The treatment is used also for patients who are over-excited, over-active and noisy, but yet feel full of energy and excessively well and do not therefore appreciate the need for rest. In order to prevent exhaustion and enable these patients to take any food or fluid at all, some form of sedation is required. Sedation, in order to take effect, may have to be somewhat heavy and prolonged. There is a danger of increased confusion and restlessness as a result of heavy sedation and if, in spite of it, the patient refuses to eat or drink and continues to be over-active, physical danger is increased rather than diminished. If a patient has been sedated for a considerable period without good results it is sometimes very much better to resort to continuous narcosis, which means really effective sedation for a limited period of time, accompanied by vigorous efforts to introduce food and fluid. Relatives often share the hospital's anxiety about the patient's physical health and will give consent to treatment when it is explained.

The Aim of Treatment

The aim of the treatment is to provide twenty hours' sleep or near sleep out of twenty-four for a period varying between ten days and three weeks. This in itself will be beneficial to some patients by breaking the habit of insomnia and the vicious circle of anxiety–insomnia–worry about insomnia–more severe insomnia.

Energy output is reduced to a minimum, and provided the food intake exceeds the basal metabolic rate, the patient will put on weight and build up some reserve which will help him if excitement or anxiety recurs at the end of the treatment. Since there may be considerable danger in the administration of large doses of possibly toxic hypnotics, very careful observation and skilled nursing care are required in order to prevent complications. The patient derives psychological benefit from the intimate and intensive nursing which he receives at the hands of a skilled, interested and understanding individual. Results achieved by this method of treatment are often more lasting and more significant than those obtained from ordinary sleep.

Preparation for Treatment

The patient should be in familiar surroundings during the treatment and should know the nurses who will be with him at the time. If possible, he should sleep the night before in the room where the treatment is to be given. He may be encouraged to write to his friends and relatives himself explaining that he should not be visited for some time and that he will be unable to write letters. If he is unable to do this, it must be done for him and he must be told that this is the case. Relatives should be encouraged to inquire by telephone and throughout the treatment the patient should be kept informed of inquiries which have been made about him, unless this is specifically contra-indicated.

A comfortable, warm, well-ventilated room is required, away from noise and free from draughts. It should be possible to darken the room and yet maintain adequate ventilation. The mattress must be soft and the bed comfortable.

The patient should have a bath before starting treatment. The bowels should be empty because constipation is likely to arise as a result of sedation and the probability of low-residue diet having to be given, and also because it may be necessary to give drugs per rectum. Temperature, pulse and respiration should be taken, because it would not be wise to begin treatment if the patient had any infective condition.

Various drugs are in use. The choice of drug for the particular patient will depend:

(1) On the drugs he has already been in the habit of taking, since these are not likely to be effective.

(2) On the patient's physical health, particularly the state of the kidneys. Drugs excreted by the kidneys may have to be avoided if the kidneys are not functioning normally. The type of drug will depend also on the patient's general condition because toxic effects may arise very rapidly if he is undernourished or dehydrated.

(3) On the doctor's preference in the light of his previous experience.

It is usual to combine two drugs, one of which is used as the basic drug and the second of which is given four-hourly if required. For example, paraldehyde may be given morning and evening and sodium amytal may be given four-hourly if necessary, or sodium amytal may be given twice daily and paraldehyde four-hourly. Soneryl or Somnifaine are other drugs used, so also are Largactil and the barbiturates, sometimes used in combination.

Tranquillizing drugs are sometimes used instead of hypnotics to produce a state of considerable relaxation. In that case it is not necessary that the patient should actually sleep for twenty hours. The nurse should be familiar with the signs to be expected in the event of the drugs giving rise to toxic effects. Dosage depends on the amount of sleep obtained, and is so arranged that the patient wakes naturally every four hours but never becomes too widely awake. If he is too over-active to accept the early doses of sedative, rectal or intravenous administration may have to be resorted to. After the first dose, however, the patient should receive further sedation while he is still drowsy and therefore more easily persuaded to accept the drug by mouth.

Nursing the Patient

One nurse on each shift should, if possible, be made responsible for the nursing of the patient and no new nurses should be introduced to him during treatment because it may be difficult for the patient to rouse himself sufficiently to identify the new person correctly. Should it become absolutely essential to have changes of nursing staff the new nurse should be introduced at length to the patient by a nurse already known to him. The nurse who will be caring for the patient during treatment should endeavour to gain his confidence beforehand, noting for example whether he has any idiosyncrasies about food, any particular likes or dislikes, and getting to know him as well as possible.

The following nursing care will be given during each twenty-four hours.

Observation of the Patient

A chart is kept, recording administration of drugs and the hours of sleep, note being taken every fifteen minutes as to whether the patient is sleeping, drowsy or wide awake. When the treatment is well on the way the dose of the drug administered will be such that the patient wakes every four hours, when a second dose should be administered. If he does not wake after four hours the nurse should wait a little, because it is better to fit in meals and nursing care with the patient's natural sleep rhythm rather than to wake him from a sound sleep. Should he not wake soon after the end of the four-hour period it is necessary to wake him in order to ensure that he can be roused and is not suffering from the effects of an overdose. Subsequent dosages will probably be reduced by the doctor until a four-hourly rhythm is established. When the patient is awake all necessary nursing care is given him as speedily and smoothly as possible, and the next dose of the drug administered while he is still drowsy.

During the short waking periods the patient is bathed or washed, his hair brushed and combed and pressure areas attended to. The bed is carefully made and during that time the patient is either helped to exercise by walking up and down with the aid of a nurse, or passive exercise of the limbs is carried out while he is in bed. Breathing exercises and changes of position will help to prevent respiratory complications. Blood circulation in the limbs is stimulated, and foot drop and contraction prevented by exercise and careful attention to posture during sleep.

Temperature, pulse, respiration and blood pressure are taken and recorded. Any evidence of cardiovascular collapse calls for immediate cessation of treatment and administration of a stimulant, which should always be in readiness, depending on the specific drug used. '

Care is needed in the administration of fluids; at least five pints should be consumed daily and the patient should be encouraged to drink whenever he is awake. A fluid balance chart should be kept, although it may be difficult to keep a strictly accurate chart because the patient may be incontinent.

Food

A nourishing, easily digested diet should be attractively prepared. The patient's drowsiness makes feeding difficult and only small meals will be acceptable. Regular urine testing should be carried out to establish that the patient is receiving sufficient food, the presence of acetone being evidence of inadequate carbohydrate intake. It may be necessary to calculate the amount of food which contains the necessary 2000 to 2500 calories in twenty-four hours. Constipation is almost inevitable and an enema may have to be administered, but this should be discussed with the doctor because he may think it inadvisable in view of the patient's fears and fantasies. A laxative may be given instead, but the disadvantage of this is that pain or discomfort may interfere with sleep.

Reassuring the Patient

The patient should never find himself alone on waking. The presence of a familiar person may be sufficient reassurance but it may be necessary for the nurse to tell him where he is and to reintroduce herself by name because the patient may mis-identify her, confusing her with someone else. It may be necessary to remind him repeatedly that he is having sleep treatment.

The patient may be restless during treatment and must be guarded against physical injury. The nurse should try to find the cause of restlessness. Very often the patient may be dreaming, and in his dream is acting out some previous experience. He may not really be asleep when he is restless, but only confused and drowsy, his restlessness being an attempt at orientating himself.

Dreams

Sometimes the patient wakes after a nightmare. Dreaming is a common occurrence during this treatment. In the early stages dreams may be similar to those which have been recurring during the neurosis or psychosis for which the patient is being treated. If the patient wakes frightened from a nightmare he is reassured if told that he has been dreaming. At the same time, if he recounts the content of his dream, an accurate note of it should be made as soon as possible for the doctor. The patient may feel happier if he is told that a record of his dreams is being kept for him, or that he can later tell his dream to the doctor if he wishes. It is not easy to remember the complicated dreams which patients tell, and they should therefore be recorded as soon as possible in the patient's exact words. No attempt should be made by the nurse to interpret the dream either to the patient or to herself before it is recorded, since this would interfere with the accuracy of the written account.

The nature of the dreams often changes during treatment. In the later stages dreams of recovery or of everyday activities may indicate the subjective experience of improvement and recovery and be a valuable guide to the doctor.

Incontinence

Because of the large amount of fluid which the patient consumes, and his state of sleep and drowsiness, he is sometimes incontinent during treatment. He may worry intensely about this, and have to be reassured that it is only to be expected and the nurse will look after him. He should be enabled to talk freely about his feelings either to the doctor or the nurse, because incontinence, and the way the patient feels about what has happened, may dominate his thoughts and may be of great importance in his treatment, depending on the fears and emotions aroused by similar situations in his childhood.

Withdrawal of Treatment

At the end of the treatment the narcotic drugs are gradually withdrawn. During withdrawal the patient may be confused or restless; the nurse should cheer him and help him to orientate himself in the ward. He will wish to be informed of all that has happened during his treatment and be brought up to date in current affairs. His letters should be read to him if he cannot himself manage to read them, and as soon as possible he should be encouraged to write home and invite visitors to come. During the withdrawal period, but also at other times during treatment, the patient may have a convulsive fit. This may be a typical *grand mal* attack, but may differ in some respects. Such fits should be observed and described in detail, noting in particular what the patient talks about when he first regains consciousness, what his wishes are, where he believes he is. The doctor should be immediately notified.

Following narcosis treatment the patient is gradually encouraged to get up and take exercise. Occupational therapy should be slowly introduced, and the patient encouraged to take an interest in his surroundings.

The intensive nursing care given during narcosis therapy is not abruptly withdrawn, but gradually diminished. The patient is very carefully encouraged to join in ward routine, the strain of social living lessened by the slow tapering off of physical treatment, and the correspondingly slow increase in the demands made upon him.

Modified Insulin Therapy

This treatment is sometimes given following continuous narcosis therapy; or it may be given as the sole measure to increase appetite and provide the patient with rest.

The patient is given an intramuscular injection of insulin as soon as he wakes in the morning. The maximal dose of insulin is administered which renders the patient drowsy but not unconscious. This is determined empirically. The patient is carefully observed throughout treatment, and prevented from passing into sopor by the timely administration of glucose by mouth. Usually a glass of fruit juice with glucose is given in the third hour of treatment followed later by breakfast with fairly high carbohydrate content.

Benefits of Therapy

Modified insulin therapy leads to increased appetite, to a gain in weight and a feeling of physical well-being. This may be highly beneficial to the patient who has been worried about tiredness and loss of appetite and has despaired of ever again feeling energetic. It may also satisfy the patient's demand for physical treatment. Some patients find it difficult to accept that their illness has psychological causes and are unwilling to co-operate with psychotherapy, demanding that some tangible physical treatment should be given. Modified insulin therapy is safe, beneficial to the patient's physical health and may give him the satisfaction of feeling that his illness is being taken seriously, and that he is receiving physical treatment which is socially acceptable. The improved relationship between psychiatrist and patient, and between nurse and patient, which develops in the course of treatment can be utilized to explore the latter's attitudes and to help in changing these. Gradually the way may be prepared for acceptance of psychotherapy if this seems desirable.

For some patients it may be important to receive extra attention. To have special treatment which no one else in the ward is receiving may be the decisive factor. More attention can be given by the nurse, without there being an appearance of favouritism or unfairness.

Other patients derive more benefit from the treatment if it is carried out in a ward where a group of patients are undergoing similar therapy. It provides some common experience, a bond which helps to make friends. It makes it possible for a number of patients to have the same daily routine and so develop a group spirit. A certain amount of discipline is necessary if insulin has been given because there is a very slight danger of hypoglycaemia. The patients as a group can submit to this discipline without losing face. They can accept dependence on a nurse without feeling uncomfortable about it; the nurse can exert authority, because it is allegedly necessary for the patient's physical safety. He may understand more readily, in these circumstances, that authority can be benign and so may be able to accept it without rebellion. This situation may prove to be the first step in establishing successful social and emotional relationships.

Many nurses find it easier to establish contact with a patient while doing something for him; they sometimes even feel uncomfortable in their relationship with patients unless there is something to do. The simple nursing procedures involved in carrying out modified insulin therapy may help patient and nurse to establish the necessary rapport for further therapy in the hospital.

PROLONGED BATHS

Prolonged baths have been used extensively in the treatment of patients who are over-active, excitable and suffering from insomnia, if for any reason it is considered inadvisable to administer large doses of sedatives.

Often during prolonged phases of excitement, the patient's physical condition gives cause for alarm. If he is losing weight and is unwilling to drink sufficient fluid the administration of heavy sedation may not be a safe procedure, while small doses of sedatives often increase restlessness and confusion. Two courses of action may then be contemplated. Either the patient may be confined in a small space and external stimulation reduced to a minimum, in the hope that excitement will subside, or attempts may be made to quieten him by the use of baths. In practice, when prolonged bathing is properly carried out, both these objectives are achieved.

It is necessary to ensure that there is no great fluctuation in the temperature of the bath and of the bathroom, in order to prevent circulatory failure, especially if the patient's physical condition is poor.

The advantage of keeping the patient in the bathroom consists in allowing him to remain undressed. Clothes often contribute considerably to his irritation. If he is over-sensitive and over-responsive to stimuli the awareness of clothes pressing or rubbing on his skin may stimulate him to tear them off. If he is repeatedly found partially or completely undressed repeated attempts have to be made to dress him again, because in an open ward, nudity, whether partial or complete, is distressing to other patients and visitors. If the patient is dressed in clothing made from strong, non-tearing material, these garments, because they are harsh and ill-fitting, increase his irritation and restlessness. The mere fact that the patient is able to remain in the nude may make nursing in the bathroom desirable.

Furthermore, it may be advisable to exclude stimulation by other patients, and in the bathroom the patient is removed from the traffic of the ward. He is unaware of the movements of people and is not in any way involved in the ward routine. He is effectively isolated from the other patients yet, unlike seclusion in his room, which he probably interprets as rejection and punishment, this isolation is achieved as a form of treatment. He is receiving special attention from the staff and is in a privileged position in relation to other patients.

Since there is no useful occupation which an excited, confused patient can successfully carry out, he is likely to become destructive. Almost any activity he may attempt will be annoying to others, or possibly dangerous to himself, and the nurses will be driven to continuous interference and will have to be excessively restrictive. Water play seems to be a possible solution to the problem. Splashing water, pouring it out and dropping things into water or just looking at water provide endless enjoyment even to healthy people and the sound of running water is immensely soothing. The patient cannot do any damage in the bath and there is no need to interfere with his activity.

All these factors contribute to the success of prolonged bath therapy, even although the actual time spent in the water may at first be quite short. The nurse usually finds it easier to 'special' the patient while he is in the bath than it would be to remain with him in his own room.

The nurse can make full use of the opportunities afforded by the continuous bath to observe the patient's preoccupations and emotions, and to record his conversation and behaviour. She can establish good rapport more easily in the atmosphere of relaxation and in a situation where she need not be restrictive.

The patient is possibly more responsive to a nurse who is with him in the bathroom for many hours and who is not wearing stiff and starchy uniform; and such a relationship, built up during hydrotherapy, can be utilized by the nurse later, when the patient is returned to the ward, in the social setting of which certain demands are again made on him.

CHAPTER 21

Malarial Therapy, Insulin Coma Therapy, Electroconvulsive Therapy, and Prefrontal Leucotomy

MALARIAL THERAPY

OF the physical treatments now in use, malarial therapy was the first. Having observed that many mentally ill patients' symptoms improve during and after physical illness, a famous psychiatrist decided to attempt to induce such an illness deliberately and then observe the mental changes which would take place. Malaria was chosen because it was an illness which could reliably be terminated when desired, and general paralysis of the insane was chosen because of the hopelessness of prognosis. A patient with this disease inevitably died within a few years and it was therefore rightly argued that any recoveries produced by malarial therapy could fairly be attributed to this treatment. It was proved that the progress of the disease could be arrested and that considerable improvement occurred in treated patients.

Malarial therapy has now been to a great extent superseded by the administration of very large doses of penicillin. The success of malarial therapy in the treatment of general paralysis of the insane led to a search for other forms of physical intervention. The use of insulin coma therapy, of electoconvulsive therapy and of prefrontal leucotomy is the outcome of this search.

INSULIN COMA THERAPY

Insulin coma therapy is now very rarely used in this country. It used to be extensively carried out in many psychiatric hospitals, with beneficial results if patients were carefully selected.

Patients who Benefit from Treatment

The patients who benefited most were those who had not been ill very long, had previously been fairly mature, well-adjusted people and whose illness was characterized by withdrawal from people and from reality. Patients who are solitary by habit and dislike all forms of social life and mixing with others are emotionally cold and therefore lack friends. These prefer to remain in their rooms, sitting in odd corners, unoccupied, disinclined to take exercise, reluctant to speak, sometimes refusing food, often neglecting their personal appearance.

With deep insulin therapy such solitarily inclined patients with schizophrenia recovered more quickly than they did with other forms of treatment. The general set-up of an insulin therapy ward lends itself very well to intensive efforts on the part of the nursing staff in establishing emotional contact with the patient and helping in his resocialization.

Extensive investigation of the effects of insulin coma therapy have now led to the conclusion that beneficial results of the treatment could not be attributed to the insulin coma itself but probably to the psychological effect of treatment.

The treatment is usually carried out in a *small* ward and this in itself may be of value to the patient. The fact that all patients are receiving the same therapy, but that some are already much improved when others are starting treatment, creates a very helpful group spirit amongst them all.

Patients who are approaching the end of treatment,

and are on the way to recovery, raise the morale of those who have newly arrived in the ward. The former can be encouraged to help the new patient and often it is easier for them than for the nursing staff to communicate with the withdrawn, apathetic, uninterested personality. The patient who is improving is helped in his rehabilitation by being useful to a weaker member of the community. Relatives also encourage each other and the patients, with the result that the atmosphere in the insulin ward is often exceptionally happy and optimistic and the most withdrawn patients are effectively brought into group relationships.

The treatment consists of inducing unconsciousness by lowering the blood sugar as a result of the injection of insulin. After a suitable duration of deep unconsciousness the patient is roused, the blood suger rising to normal after the administration of glucose.

While the patient undergoes therapy, he receives, as early as possible every morning, an intramuscular injection of insulin. The first day, a very small dose is given, and no reaction is anticipated. If a reaction to a very small dose were to occur the patient would not continue with treatment.

The dose of insulin is usually increased until a degree of unconsciousness termed 'coma' is reached in the third hour after administration of insulin. This dose is maintained daily, or possibly slightly reduced, until thirty or forty comas have been given.

Insulin treatment, even in skilled hands, is potentially dangerous and it is very unpleasant to the patient. As there is no evidence that the insulin coma in itself is in any way beneficial it is now generally believed that the social and psychological benefits accompanying the treatment can be provided more directly by other treatment approaches.

ELECTROCONVULSIVE THERAPY

Electroconvulsive therapy is a technically simple treatment, but the patient requires support and reassurance from tactful and understanding nursing staff.

It is a treatment which, because it is relatively safe, quick, cheap and frequently effective, has been used somewhat indiscriminately in recent years. It has been employed in out-patient departments, clinics and hospitals, and has proved beneficial in a variety of mental disorders.

One of the results of its very widespread use is that it is now rare to meet a patient who has never heard of this form of treatment. Most patients have known someone, or heard of someone who has been treated with ' E.C.T.'. The patient's attitude is therefore coloured by the experience of his friends. He will eagerly demand this treatment if he knows of someone who was cured, or fear it if his experience has been unfavourable. He may have heard accounts of the treatment from someone who had unmodified convulsive therapy and therefore dread the discomfort associated with it. He may also fear that his condition must be as bad as that of someone else he has known if the same treatment is recommended. There is a tendency to assume that similar treatments can only be prescribed for those having similar disorders.

Even if the patient has not heard of electroconvulsive therapy prior to admission he will almost certainly meet in hospital those who are undergoing this treatment. Patients can often be heard discussing their treatment with each other and comparing notes, and the nurse can easily discover how the patient is likely to react to the news that he is to have electroconvulsive therapy by observing him while other patients talk about it.

The Patient's Fears

Consent from patient and relatives is often required. Explaining treatment to the patient is difficult unless a good deal is known about his particular fears and worries and the doctor who has to do this will appreciate any helpful information. After the doctor has explained the treatment to the patient, the nurse is often approached by the patient, who asks questions about it, hoping to have the doctor's words confirmed. The nurse must find out from the doctor what explanation he has given, and she must ask the patient what the doctor has said. Nothing could be worse for the patient than apparent contradiction between doctor and nurses. Nurses should agree in their approach to the patient, since the more contradictory information he receives, the more people he will approach for reassurance.

The line taken by the doctor depends on the patient's anticipation. Sometimes he stresses the fact that there is no pain or discomfort and that the patient will remember nothing about it. But this is the very thing which some patients worry about, if they happen to have heard about the loss of memory which follows E.C.T. In this case the doctor will assure the patient that loss of memory is only transitory and that there is no danger of important things being forgotten.

Some patients are afraid of the possible pain or danger of the treatment. Others demand electroconvulsive therapy because they believe that the very nature of this drastic treatment will help, or even because feelings of guilt and unworthiness cause them to regard it as something in the nature of deserved punishment. It would be little reassurance for such patients to be told that the treatment is quite harmless.

There is so far no satisfactory name for the treatment which could be used in talking to the patients. Abbreviations such as 'E.C.T.' are not very helpful because the patient demands explanation. 'Electro' is a terrifying word to many patients. Many delusional systems include the idea of the use of electricity on the brain or the influence of electricity on thought processes. It is not at all pleasant to think of electricity being applied to the brain in a manner which the patient himself cannot understand or observe. On the other hand some patients believe that there exists some magical influence which is associated with the use of electricity and feel sure that 'electrical treatment' will cure them.

The word 'convulsive' for those who understand it, does nothing to mitigate their horror of electricity, so it is better avoided. This leaves 'shock' therapy, again an unfortunate expression to use.

Many nurses avoid the dilemma by talking simply about 'treatment', even using the plural 'treatments'. This has the unfortunate effect that the patient talks about having had '6 treatments' when really he may have had six convulsions in the course of six months' treatment. It tends to make the patients feel that E.C.T. only *is* 'treatment', and makes it more difficult to place proper emphasis on environmental and psychological influences. This results in patients who are discharged well (after a few months of intensive therapy from psychiatrists, nurses, social workers and occupational therapists) telling their relatives that they have received no treatment at all.

Preparing the Patient for Treatment

However carefully the patient is prepared, on the day of his first E.C.T. he will experience a great deal of fear and apprehension, which the nurse must try to alleviate. It is usual for the patients to have little or no breakfast on the day of treatment, which makes it inevitable that E.C.T. should be preceded by anxious anticipation. It is difficult for the patient to be occupied until the last moment if he is fasting and has to remain in bed. The best thing is to tell him at approximately what time he will be having treatment and to attempt to be as punctual as possible. The worst of the waiting time occurs after the original appointment.

If no muscle relaxant is given the patient requires no further preparation except to remove tight clothing, dentures, hairpins and to empty his bladder, all these at the last possible moment. The patient is fully conscious while the apparatus is being prepared and while he is being placed in position, so that no conversation should take place which is not addressed to him personally. A commentary and explanation of what is happening is given.

Sometimes E.C.T. is carried out in one central place to which all patients are taken. At other hospitals the machine is taken to the patient. Whichever arrangement is adopted, some attention must be paid to the layout of the ward, so that patients who are waiting do not see or hear any of the patients who have had shock treatments, because these are sometimes noisy on waking. Any trolleys with syringes, oxygen apparatus or any other equipment should be kept out of sight, and only the shortest possible time should be spent waiting. While waiting a nurse should always be present, guiding conversation and providing distraction from the topic of E.C.T.

During electroconvulsive therapy without modification a certain amount of restraint is sometimes required. A small pillow or sandbag is usually placed in the lumbar region of the spine and light pressure on shoulders and hips should prevent injury. The most important duty of the nurses concerned is to estimate each other's strength and to supply pressure evenly on both sides. This can be practised on a colleague and will prevent discomfort and injury to the patient.

After Treatment

Following E.C.T. the patient gradually returns to consciousness and requires a familiar face and familiar voice near him. He will be confused, not knowing where he is or how he arrived there and will certainly not remember having had E.C.T. It may be necessary to speak slowly but clearly, in short sentences, re-introducing the patient in concrete terms to the people and objects around him, naming objects used, e.g. cup, spoon, bed, blanket; using the patient's name when addressing him. The nurse should mention her own name, or that of any other nurse. It saves embarrassment and worry to say 'Nurse Smith will give you a cup of tea' rather than to leave the patient to try and remember Nurse Smith's name, by merely referring to her as 'Nurse'.

For some hours after E.C.T. the patient may have difficulty in remembering and to many patients this is very worrying. Over and over again the patient may approach the nurse and ask the question. 'This is Thursday, isn't it?', or 'Is it supper-time yet, nurse?', or 'Is this my bed?' Time and time again the patient tries to reorientate himself in the ward and, so long as he is not snubbed, he comes to the nurse for confirmation that he remembers correctly. He needs reassurance that this is only a temporary side effect of the treatment, and outweighed by the fact that he 'feels so much better'. Careful observation during the confused period is necessary because the patient may enter someone else's bed, use someone else's belongings or wander off through any doors accidentally left open, possibly even out into the road, where he might meet with an accident. Not until the patient has fully recovered his orientation can he be safely left out of sight.

Administration of Muscle Relaxants

Should E.C.T. be given with a muscle relaxant, e.g. Brevidil-M or Scoline, there will be less need for re-straint during the fit because muscle spasm is consider-ably reduced. The patient has an intravenous anaes-thetic, e.g. Pentothal, at the same time as, or a few moments before, the muscle relaxant, so that he does not feel the gradual paralysis. There is less fear of treatment and therefore less need for keeping the patients away from each other before treatment. Because the patient is given atropine before leaving the ward he will complain of thirst and a certain amount of anxiety may be present. After the fit the patient requires oxygen and artificial respiration making sure the airway is clear.

Complications after E.T.C. are rare, provided the patient has been carefully observed prior to the anaesthetic and has undergone a thorough physical examination.

Because his muscles are relaxed the patient's position on the bed or trolley during the treatment must be carefully observed to guard against injury and deformity. A special mouthgag is used to prevent biting of the tongue. The distribution of the patient's teeth determines the most suitable shape of airway and mouthgag, for a tooth might break if the patient were to bite too forcibly on a hard part of the gag. The electrodes which are placed on the patient's forehead are padded and soaked in hypertonic saline or other electrolyte fluid and must be kept wet to prevent burns. Recovery is usually fairly rapid, but the patient must be as carefully guarded against accidents during the confused period, as when E.C.T. is given unmodified.

Behaviour after Treatment

The patient's mood and behaviour undergoes considerable change during the course of convulsive treatments which should be carefully observed and reported. Usually, after the first few shocks, the patient becomes brighter, more active and his appetite and physical condition improve. Occasionally, as he becomes more active, more able to think and act, has more energy, moves faster, he is more able than before to put into practice any suicidal plans he has made during his more retarded period. Vigilance should not be relaxed until the thought content, as well as the mood, has ceased to be depressive.

Sometimes when the depression lifts, and the patient is more able to express his thoughts in words, it becomes evident that a severe thought disorder is present and that depression was not the only symptom. The period between convulsive treatments may well be the most fruitful time for establishing contact with a patient who as a rule is disinclined to talk, and may be the time when, with the help of observant nursing staff, a more accurate diagnosis can be made.

Any improvement shown by the patient should be fully utilized by the nursing staff, not only in raising his morale, but in attending to any physical symptoms which may be present, increasing food intake, providing exercise and generally building up the physical condition. Contact with relatives can be re-established and the patient can be helped to form satisfying social relationships with other patients in the hospital, so that, even if improvement is not permanent or recovery complete, he will still be in a better position to cope with a long illness than would otherwise have been the case.

PREFRONTAL LEUCOTOMY

Brain surgery as a form of treatment in mental illness has been introduced only comparatively recently and although the number of patients treated by one form or another of brain surgery is now considerable, and the literature on the subject extensive, knowledge of the effects of the treatment is still limited. Various techniques in severing association fibres from the frontal lobes to the thalamus are practised by surgeons in this and other countries, and there is general agreement that some patients have derived considerable benefit. It is, however, too early to say which patients benefit most and which operation offers the greatest hope for a favourable prognosis in individual cases.

Although so little is known about the effects of the

treatment there is a great deal of controversy both among doctors and among the general public regarding the ethical implications of carrying out a drastic operation of uncertain value, which is irreversible and in some cases accompanied by undesirable side effects. In many cases, however, the beneficial results far outweigh the less desirable consequences. Some doctors feel that only in patients where prognosis is utterly hopeless and where all other forms of treatment have failed is surgical intervention justifiable. Others argue that prognosis is better if early intervention takes place and advocate better selection of suitable patients for operation.

Results depend so much on the selection of suitable patients, and on their aftercare and rehabilitation, that the nurse plays a vital part in furthering knowledge. At present doctors find it difficult to compare results because information about the patient's prepsychotic personality, the character of the illness and the method of pre- and post-operative care is scanty and may be unreliable. The nurse can help to supply this information, which will contribute materially to the future development of surgery in psychiatry.

The patient's view is usually taken into account. The operation is hardly ever carried out without specific consent from himself and his relatives. The doctor explains the treatment to the patient and tries to allay existing fears. The nurse must support whatever arguments the doctor has used in favour of treatment and never allow her own prejudices, if she has any, to influence the patient.

The operation is usually preceded by extensive and prolonged investigations. The fact that the patient is not rushed into treatment, but that the decision to advise operation is made after due consideration of all relevant facts, is reassuring both to him and his relatives.

Relatives and patients usually wish to know what changes are likely to occur in the patient's personality.

This question is difficult to answer because of the wide variability which has been observed. It would be wise to say that some patients have recovered completely without any detriment to previous personality, without, however, implying that this will necessarily be the outcome in any particular case.

Modern neurosurgical techniques have reduced the severity of personality changes, and have made it easier to predict what changes to expect. In order to establish what changes have taken place it is necessary to compare the patient's pre- and post-operative behaviour in comparable situations. Full observation of the patient's behaviour in specific situations is necessary, and a detailed record should be made before, and again after, the operation. His reaction to frustrating situations in the ward are of importance and it should always be made clear, not only how he behaved but how, and with what results, the nurse tried to deal with the situation.

Outcome of the Operation

Leucotomy may be performed on patients whose life is made intolerable by persistent hallucinations or by incapacitating obsessional rituals. Following the operation hallucinations may persist, but they may no longer worry the patient. Obsessional rituals may continue, but the patient no longer responds with agonizing anxiety when the rituals are interrupted.

Personality Changes after Leucotomy

It appears that the following personality changes take place fairly frequently:

Intelligence as measured by intelligence tests is unimpaired. The most striking changes are emotional ones and the operation is usually performed in order to relieve the patient of the intolerable emotional tension from which he suffers. But the emotional blunting which takes place may not be entirely beneficial. The patient may become indifferent not only to his own compulsive, ruminative or delusional thoughts, but also to the thoughts and feelings of others. He may become less responsive than before to love, affection and friendship, less aware of other people's emotional reactions to his own behaviour and so appear to be self-centred, unconcerned and tactless. The extent to which his conduct may be impaired depends on the extent to which his behaviour was ruled by habit, social convention or emotional factors.

The most serious ill-effects may arise where the patient's tension has resulted from an endeavour to keep violent and antisocial impulses under control. Removing emotional control from such a patient might well enable him to indulge in antisocial behaviour without any feeling of guilt or worry. However, very few antisocial acts of this nature have been reported and better observation before operation should help to identify those patients who are likely to become aggressive after surgery has been performed.

Apathy may become the patient's most serious handicap but it should be possible to overcome this with carefully planned and skilfully conducted post-operative training.

Pre-operative Care

The immediate pre-operative care is very simple once the patient's consent for operation is obtained and he is able to accept the treatment.

Skin preparation varies. Some surgeons like to adhere to repeated shaving and cleansing of scalp, as for other bone operations. Others, however, leave shaving until the last possible moment and do not require any form of skin preparation, other than shampoo of the head. They argue that minor cuts or abrasions are inevitable in shaving and the less the risk of infection due to the presence of these cuts the better.

Psychologically it is better for the patient to be shaved

as late as possible, since he does not usually like to be seen by his fellow patients after his hair is shaved. Some surgeons wish to see the entire head shaved; others agree to the shaving of only a small area of the patient's scalp.

To a female patient it is usually comforting to know that only part of the hair will be cut and the nurses should promise that every effort will be made by skilled hairdressing to arrange the remaining hair in an attractive hair style. Patients have at times expressed the wish, if the hair is long, to have a wig made of their own hair; strands of hair should therefore be cut with the greatest possible care.

Some sedation is probably ordered to ensure a good night's rest prior to operation. Premedication depends on the anaesthetic to be used, which is frequently only a local one.

The patient has a light diet on the day prior to operation, and the last meal should be taken no later than four hours before operation. Fluids may be restricted as a means of reducing intracranial pressure.

The patient should not be constipated and a thorough physical examination and urine analysis are carried out on the eve of the operation.

The patient is taken to the operating theatre by a nurse whom the patient knows and trusts, preferably the nurse who has attended to the last-minute preparations, e.g. emptying of bladder, covering of hair, removal of dentures, changing into a warm gown. The nurse should remain in the theatre and be present when the patient recovers consciousness. Her voice will help him to re-orientate himself when he wakes in the theatre, as it is usual to keep the patient on the operating table until he is fully conscious.

Post-operative Care

During the first few hours after operation the observation of pulse and respiration is important in order to enable detection to be made immediately in the event of haemorrhage and raised intracranial pressure. The patient is kept in bed and the nurse reports whether the state of consciousness is improving or regressing, whether there are any abnormal movements, e.g. twitching or convulsion. Pupil reaction, eye movements, speech and facial movements are observed.

Very little fluid is given during the first twenty-four hours and then only if the patient is not vomiting. It may be desirable to pass a stomach tube and aspirate the contents of the stomach in order to spare the patient the effort involved in vomiting, an effort liable to increase intracranial pressure.

A hypertonic magnesium sulphate enema may be ordered several times following the operation if oedema of the brain is still present. Careful attention to the mouth is required because fluid intake is restricted. Urine output should be measured and some efforts made to ensure that the patient passes urine within twelve hours after operation. Some sedation is usually required in order to prevent restlessness, but morphine is never used after intracranial surgery. The dressing is usually left intact until the stitches are removed, usually on about the seventh day.

The patient may remain in bed for about a week, and during that time he will receive the usual nursing care, with encouragement of gradually increasing independence.

Confusional symptoms commonly occur, and provided the patient is guarded against injury they are not considered as serious complications. The nurse helps the patient during confused periods by speaking slowly, clearly and audibly, avoiding unnecessary chatter, whispering and noise. Unless the patient complains of photophobia, it is usually better, in order to avoid shadows, to keep lights on rather than subdued. Unnecessary changes in nursing staff are avoided. The fluid balance is carefully recorded.

Excessive restlessness and any unexpected complications, e.g. rise in temperature, sudden changes in rate and volume of pulse or changes in blood pressure, must be reported at once.

Post-operative Rehabilitation

Early ambulation is advisable, and if no complications occur after about a week post-operative rehabilitation begins. This depends on the end results which are hoped for or expected. These differ in the case of the patient who has spent many years in a psychiatric hospital, in a state of complete degradation, and who, it is hoped, will be helped to become a useful if somewhat docile member of the chronic psychiatric hospital community, and in that of a patient who is to return to a full and active life in the larger community outside.

It is very necessary to be clear before the operation is performed what kind of improvement would appear satisfactory to the patient, relatives and hospital and to plan in detail how the rehabilitation towards this goal is to be carried out. All those concerned, doctors, nurses, occupational therapists, social workers, the patient and his family, should be aware of the aim and should co-ordinate their efforts. As rehabilitation progresses all the staff should periodically evaluate their efforts, try to assess the patient's progress, and should endeavour to keep an accurate record of the part they themselves are playing in keeping him active and stimulated. Not only should they report what they are doing for him, but also how they are setting about their task and how much effort is involved before a response is obtained.

Progress should also be assessed by someone who does not know the patient at all, who therefore does not experience any personal sense of success or failure as a result of his behaviour. Clinical psychologists, for instance, can help considerably by administration of psychological tests before and at intervals after operation.

The patient's closest relatives are better able than the hospital staff to assess some aspects of his progress. His behaviour at home is so well known to them that they notice minor changes which are not observed in the hospital.

In order to be successful in rehabilitation each nurse must be firmly convinced that her personal contribution can be of utmost importance to the patient's recovery. Each nurse is therefore tempted to see improvement where it may not really exist. If she is not very careful, she may be selective in her reporting, so that the more favourable aspects of the patient's behaviour are noticed and reported early, the more unfavourable ones later as time passes.

She can guard against this to a certain extent by keeping behaviour charts which give a picture of the patient over long periods, instead of high-lighting any particular incident. She can also give minutely detailed accounts of particular situations on repeated occasions so that behaviour in similar circumstances can be compared.

Certain stages in rehabilitation are usually followed. At first, regular toilet habits are encouraged and the nurse may feel satisfied if the patient succeeds in dressing himself, remaining well-groomed throughout the day and attending to his own toilet at regular intervals. Next an attempt is to be made to help the patient to partake of communal meals. Table manners require supervision and constant reminders may be necessary. Patients sometimes have voracious appetites following leucotomy and must of course be prevented from hoarding food or snatching it from other patients' plates, so depriving the latter of their fair share.

The next step in rehabilitation involves occupation, and the patient is gradually encouraged to occupy himself for longer periods and at increasingly complex tasks. The last stage of rehabilitation involves the patient's home and family and his complete social and economic readjustment in his own social setting.

How each stage of rehabilitation is managed, varies with every patient. A few general principles may be stated.

If the patient is at all likely to return home and take up his old employment, he should aim at doing so in the shortest possible time. Trying to adjust to a return to home and to daily work after a prolonged period of absence is always difficult even for people who have not been ill. Changes take place all the time in all social settings, and the patient will have greater difficulties in readjusting if he finds that not only he himself but everything around him has changed, so that all his previously successful methods of adaptation have become useless.

A very important point to remember at all times is that most patients' capacity for relearning old, forgotten skills and learning new ones is very great indeed, and that it can proceed for a very long time. Progress may continue for many years following operation and hope should never be abandoned. Learning takes place only if the patient is adequately motivated to learn and if appropriate methods of teaching are used. At each stage, the nurse must decide what she would like the patient to learn and help him to do the right and not the wrong thing. At each stage she must make it clear to the patient what is required of him and why the particular behaviour is thought to be desirable.

The patient is helped in learning by practice and repetition and by being kept informed of his progress. He is helped by approval when he is successful and by reminders when he is not. Prior to operation repeated correction of the patient's behaviour may have been deeply resented and he may have become angry, abusive and perhaps violent, or have cut off his relationship with the nurse in such a way that further teaching may have become impossible. After the operation the patient is less likely to react violently to the nurse's attempt at retraining, and success is much more likely to be achieved.

The patient cannot learn if too much is expected of him at once. Each new skill must be introduced carefully and singly.

The great majority of patients will acquire competence at some occupation and will successfully manage their own life within the simple, ordered routine and sheltered atmosphere of a psychiatric hospital.

Greater difficulties will be encountered in helping patients to regain their social skills and in encouraging initiative. Many patients remain apathetic and permanently need somebody who can take the initiative for them. Very often the patient's relatives are prepared to accept this role if it is explained to them. If the patient goes home for increasing periods of time, returning to the hospital several times before finally being discharged home, he and his relatives are able to learn how to live successfully with each other.

CHAPTER 22

The Use of Drugs

In the last two decades the introduction of new drugs has transformed psychiatric treatment.

Much research is going on in all countries into the effect of new drugs on the function of the nervous system. The fact that some drugs are found to have specific effects on certain psychological processes has given impetus to research into the nature of mental illness itself. Some drugs, for example, cause hallucinations, others have specific use in diminishing hallucinations. It seems logical to link research into the effect of such drugs with research into the causation of hallucinations.

Some drugs have specifically beneficial results in states of depression, others in manic excitement. This knowledge leads to research into the chemical changes taking place in depressive or manic states, and into the possibility of biochemical causation of these disorders.

While some drugs are used for their specific effect, others are used for their general sedating or stimulating effect. Some psychiatrists are interested chiefly in the specific action of drugs they use. Other psychiatrists regard social and psychological methods of treatment as more important. They readily agree, however, that patients who are excessively anxious or disturbed are not amenable to psychotherapy or to sociotherapeutic influences. They use drugs to enable the patient to participate more fully in the activities of the hospital.

Drug treatment, more than other forms of physical treatment, is based on scientific research. Such research is only possible with knowledgeable contributions from nursing staff. Prescription of drugs is dependent on reliable observation of patient's behaviour and accurate reporting of change of behaviour.

Research into the effect of drugs is initially carried out on animals. When a drug has been found safe for use on human beings, drug trials are necessary to establish what effect, if any, the drug has on patients.

It is necessary to find a group of patients all of whom have a particular set of symptoms and who could be expected to benefit from the drug if the claims made for it were found to be true. Detailed reports must be available for all these patients as regards the history of the illness, the severity of the symptoms and the degree of incapacity. A careful record must be kept of all the therapeutic influences brought to bear and the patient's reaction to them. Some of the patients are then given the drug while the remainder of the group are treated in exactly the same manner in every respect except that the drug is withheld. Progress is carefully recorded over a considerable period.

This is the pattern employed in every trial of a new drug, and an attempt is always made as far as possible to match the two groups, so that the difference in result can be fairly attributed to the drug, rather than to other factors, e.g. age, differences in the duration or severity of illness, or differences in treatment other than the drug itself.

In psychiatric treatment it is particularly difficult to control the general treatment of patients, and it is here that the nurse's observations and accurate reporting can make all the difference when results are compared.

It must be taken into account that the giving of a drug may have a considerable significance for the patient. The very fact that the doctor has prescribed a drug for him may convince him that something is being done to help him. He may feel that the doctors have discovered the real cause of his trouble. He may believe that only if the cause of the trouble is known can a remedy in the form of a drug be given. The patient may also believe that this cause is physical, since it appears reasonable to him that a physical disorder should receive drug therapy. To a certain extent this may make him feel that his complaint is more 'respectable', that it can be talked about like other illnesses.

There are usually certain physiological effects, e.g. palpitations or increased pulse rate, observable both to the patient and the nurses. The patient may observe himself closely once he realizes these manifestations. He may discover signs and symptoms in himself which he had not previously noticed but which he now interprets as changes in the course of his illness.

Nurses, having been warned of the possible ill-effects of the drug, observe the patient more carefully and with greater concern and this closer relationship between the patient and his nurse may have some beneficial effect on him.

All this may mean that the actual administration of a drug introduces a significant difference in the treatment of the patients. It is, therefore, the usual practice to give all patients some drug—a placebo to one group and the drug to be tested to the other group. Sometimes the drug is dispensed by the pharmacist in such a form that neither the nurse nor the doctor knows which patients receive the drug and which patients the placebo. Changes can be made later, the patients who have received the drug can be given the placebo without their own knowledge or the knowledge of the nurses.

The doctors' and nurses' reports can then be independently assessed and some progress made in the proper use of drugs for the patient most likely to benefit.

Some nurses feel guilty about their part in drug trials.

It is generally understood that honesty and truthfulness are the correct approach to the patient, so that the administration of a placebo appears deceitful. Occasionally it seems unkind to deprive the patient of the drug which might help him and to allow his symptoms to continue while administering only a placebo. It must, however, be remembered that mental disorders very frequently remit without specific treatment, and that the psychological significance of taking tablets is very great.

Extravagant claims are frequently made for new drugs, which later turn out to have been quite unwarranted. To protect patients from possible harmful effects and to ensure that systematic knowledge of the effect of drugs on different mental disorder is obtained, controlled drug trials are indispensable. No patient is ever submitted to harmful treatment and doctors will see to it that no patient is deprived for long of the best available form of treatment.

If the nurse conveys to the patient that she feels dubious about the pill she is offering she is not only hindering progress but also depriving the patient of the benefit which derives from an enthusiastic and positive approach.

ADMINISTRATION OF DRUGS

Whatever the drug in use, it is the nurse's duty, as soon as it has been ordered, to acquaint herself with all that is known about its action and potentialities.

She must know:

(1) The prescribed dose, and the maximal dose that can be given.
(2) The method of administration and any special points arising from it.
(3) The expected effects of the drug.
(4) The side-effects which can occur.
(4) The possible ill-effects it may produce.

The nurse is responsible for the safe keeping and storage of the drug. When administering a drug to a mental patient she should remember that identification of the patient may present more difficulties than in the case of patients in general hospitals, since the former himself may be incapable of confirming his name and unable to remember that he is having any medicine.

SEDATIVES

Sedatives are liberally used in psychiatry. This is understandable when it is remembered that insomnia is a common symptom in many mental disorders, and that sedation is also frequently required in the daytime in order to overcome anxiety, restlessness and excitement, which are exhausting to the patient.

Sedation is always ordered by the doctor and never administered by the nurse without a prescription in writing. The doctor bases his prescription on a number of factors. He takes into consideration the patient's complaints and wishes concerning sedation. He requires the nurse's report on the patient's behaviour during day and night. The patient's physical condition determines the choice of sedatives.

Skill, tact and ability on the part of the nursing staff are essential when heavy sedation is required. As prescribed by a skilled physician and properly administered, sedatives are perfectly safe and there is no reason why prolonged sedation should not be undertaken.

Many nurses find it difficult to regard as objectively the administration of sedatives as that of other drugs. Like many other people, they may hold very strong views about sedation, believing that it is wrong to take sedatives and that it is their duty to give out as few of these as possible. Some nurses, however, may take the opposite view and think that their work is made unnecessarily difficult if the physicians are reluctant to prescribe sedation.

Patients often have strong bias against taking sedatives when these would be beneficial: or they may demand sedation without allowing time to see if sleep is possible without the help of drugs. The result of these strong emotional reactions to the administration of sedatives is that overt arguments or hidden tensions may arise and then militate against any beneficial results of these drugs.

Unnecessary Sedation

In some psychiatric hospitals the staff are proud of the fact that they have been able greatly to reduce the administration of sedatives, and they have good reason to be pleased. They point to wards full of chronic patients who in the past had been heavily sedated and who now, happily occupied during the day, sleep well at night without sedation. These patients had obviously formerly been unnecessarily sedated. Often, as a result of sedation, usually paraldehyde, the patients were confused, restless and noisy during the day, yet too drowsy and tired to be properly occupied. Then at night they were not tired, having done nothing all day. If they did not sleep they were again sedated so that they were again drowsy and confused in the morning. If sedatives are dispensed with during the day, the patients can be out of doors for exercise. They can be usefully employed and are lively, much happier and much more contented. Provided they do not go to bed too early and have the necessary physical comfort in bed, patients should have several hours' undisturbed sleep without sedation.

The position is quite different in the case of acutely disturbed psychotic or neurotic patients. Sedation will almost certainly be required and prescribed. A reason for deliberately withholding sedatives might be that some patients receiving psychotherapy are more ready to discuss their problems after a restless night of worry, dreams and nightmares than after a night of heavily sedated sleep. The doctor may then obtain the patient's consent in trying to forego narcotics. The nurse must be informed if this is the case, because a patient who is not sleeping will require more support from her.

Types of Sedatives

The sedatives which are commonly used fall into two groups:

(a) Those which are believed to act quickly but for brief periods only;

(b) those which are believed to have prolonged but not immediate action.

Sodium Amytal, Seconal, Nembutal and Soneryl are examples of drugs in the first group. Phenobarbitone and Medinal belong to the second group. Some patients react differently to these drugs, so that a strict classification into slow and quick acting sedatives is not possible.

The drugs prescribed for any individual patient depend on his personal idiosyncrasies, on the drugs he had been having before, on the doctor's preference, based on past experience, and on the patient's sleep rhythm as reported by the nurse.

Nursing Sedated Patients

The nurse should keep a regular half-hourly check on the sleep of her patients and report not only how many hours' sleep each has had, but mention when there has been interrupted sleep, restlessness, late settling down or early waking.

Slowly acting sedatives should be given out some time before the patients retire to bed, whereas those which have rapid effects but are short-acting should not be administered until the patients are settled and ready to go to sleep, because otherwise the effects will have worn off before the patient can feel peaceful enough to sleep.

If the patient is trying to sleep without sedation but a drug is written up to be given 'if required', a quick-acting drug must be used. Similarly, any drug to be repeated must be of a quick-acting variety.

In hospital it is most difficult to provide a night long enough to allow for the proper action of sedatives. It is obviously undesirable to turn out lights too soon. Hospital patients should lead as normal a life as possible and this should include fairly normal bedtime. If lights are switched off too early patients are not tired, they toss and turn, become uncomfortable and have a poor night's sleep.

If the lights are switched off, say, at 10 p.m., or later, one hour at least should be allowed, perhaps longer, before sedatives are administered which are only to be administered if required. These will be given out between 11 p.m. and midnight, and repeat sedatives not before 2 a.m. or 3 a.m. This makes it imperative, if drug hang-over effects are to be avoided, that patients should not be roused in the morning before 7 a.m. or 8 a.m.

The nurse's report on sleep is most important if the most appropriate sedation is to be prescribed. It is essential that all arguments about sleep should be avoided. The doctor often asks the patient how he has slept and, regardless of the nurse's report, accepts the statement that he has not slept a wink as an indication that the patient is not satisfied with the sleep he is having. It is useless to become angry if the patient says he has not slept when the nurse knows that he has. Even very short wakeful periods seem very long to those lying awake and the nurse only intermittently observes the patient. It is not always possible to be certain that a patient is sleeping; he may be awake without showing it. What matters is the way the patient feels about his sleep. A sleepless night is of no consequence if the patient does not mind, whereas a short period of insomnia is serious to one who is anxious and worried.

When a drug has been prescribed 'if required' some discussion is necessary to determine who should decide when repeated administration becomes necessary. The patient may be the best person to consult. He knows when he is feeling tense, and often a small amount of sedative taken before the patient's panic mounts may be effective, while if the patient had to wait longer sedatives may no longer work.

Nurses may believe that they are in fact the best judges as to when is the right time for the administration of sedatives, but it must be remembered that a patient who feels that he must fight for his sedative, and that he may not receive it unless he proves his case, is liable to develop increasingly disturbed behaviour and must eventually be given a drug. If the patient's co-operation can be obtained and he understands clearly that he must allow a safe period, for example 4 hours, to elapse before the drug can be repeated, it is usually best for him to take responsibility for making the decision to sleep without or with sedative.

Many anxious patients sleep better at night if they have a small dose of a slow-acting sedative throughout the day and a quick-acting one is administered at night.

Although most sedatives are safe the nurse should bear in mind that cumulative action is possible, and that the rate of excretion and toxicity of the drug depend on a healthy state of the liver and kidney. Urine should be tested regularly, and the patient should have adequate intake of carbohydrates and fluid. If bromides are administered, salt included in the diet aids excretion and the blood bromide level is estimated periodically, especially if confusion or excitement increases or if a rash appears. Paraldehyde, because it is excreted by the lungs, is often prescribed if barbiturates appear contra-indicated, but the unpleasant taste and smell are a disadvantage.

STIMULANTS

Stimulant drugs such as Benzedrine, ephedrine, Dexedrine and Methedrine, have been used in the treatment of a variety of disorders. In many patients their administration causes a sense of well-being, an increase in energy which helps a hospital patient to derive more benefit from other therapeutic measures, e.g. occupational therapy and social and recreational therapy. Depressed patients are often less retarded after the administration of stimulants and therefore less inclined to suffer from the secondary effects of inactivity. On the other hand, unless the patient also feels less depressed, there is increased danger of suicide.

Benzedrine has a very marked effect on some children and adults with behaviour disorders characterized by restlessness, irritability, temper tantrums. These patients often have abnormal electrical discharges of the brain. They tolerate Benzedrine in quite large doses and, unlike other people, become quieter rather than more active after its administration.

All these drugs have some effect on the autonomic nervous system, sometimes causing a rise in blood pressure, loss of appetite, insomnia, palpitations and tremors. The nurse should look out for undesirable side effects without, however, suggesting them to the patient. The drug may have to be discontinued, or the dose modified if complications occur.

HORMONES

The thyroid gland plays a very important part in maintaining balanced metabolism. Many psychiatrists believe that certain psychiatric disorders are associated with some metabolic dysfunction, although how this happens has not yet been explained. It is, however, known that some patients who have recurrent attacks of disorders resembling catatonic excitement or stupor respond well to regular administration of thyroid extract and a diet in which nitrogen is controlled. Some patients seem to tolerate large doses of thyroid extract and to benefit from it.

So far, very little is known about the effect of endocrine or other biochemical disturbance on mental processes. Much research is now in progress which may eventually lead to more accurate diagnosis based on clinical and pathological findings and to the rational use of drugs for specific disorder.

To obtain the necessary information it is essential not only to carry out detailed metabolic investigation on large numbers of patients, but also to accompany laboratory findings by equally reliable and detailed information from the nursing staff about the patients' behaviour, mood and speech.

TRANQUILLIZERS

These are a group of drugs which produce a calming effect without at the same time causing drowsiness or acting as hypnotics. When these drugs were introduced into psychiatric hospitals they produced dramatic effects and hope was expressed that some hitherto intractable and chronic conditions might be cured.

The beneficial results of these drugs are manifold. Because patients are calm and quiet the ward atmosphere has in many cases improved. Struggles and restraint are avoided. It is easier to establish active programmes of habit training, occupational therapy, rehabilitation and to built up relationships of trust between patients and nurses which help in later treatment.

Extensive research has resulted in so many drugs now being on the market that no details can usefully be given. All the drugs produce some unpleasant side effects and all are toxic to a greater or lesser extent. Research has been directed to finding those drugs which have the most specific therapeutic effects and the lowest degree of toxicity. Most drugs are produced by more than one firm under different trade names. It would be futile to attempt to learn the details of all of these. When the doctor prescribes a drug which is new to the nurse she should request from the pharmacist the relevant information and ensure that she memorizes the essential facts about the drug for as long as it is in use.

The main groups of tranquillizing drugs at present in use are, chemically:

(1) Phenothiazine derivatives of which chloropromazine (Largactil) is an example.

(2) Reserpine and its derivatives.

(3) Drugs of other chemical composition including Librium and Equanil and haloperidol.

The effects of these drugs fall into two categories.

(1) There are some drugs which act mainly as tranquillizers in a general way.

(2) Some drugs have more marked effect on delusions and hallucinations.

Tranquillizers are used in the treatment of patients suffering from alcoholism and drug addiction, to alleviate withdrawal symptoms and control agitation and restlessness.

All these drugs are prescribed in very large doses in order to produce therapeutic effects. Side effects are therefore common. These include such symptoms as increased appetite and gain in weight, nasal stuffiness, sore throat, dry mouth, facial rash occurring particularly when the skin is exposed to sunshine. A more serious side effect is fainting due to sudden fall in blood pressure. Unexplained pyrexia occurs in some patients; jaundice sometimes occurs when Largactil is used. Some of the side effects are neurological. Some patients complain of stiffness of limbs, pain and a peculiar restlessness and jitteriness. Parkinsonian signs may develop and these are treated with anti-Parkinsonian drugs such as Disipal. Agranulocytosis occasionally occurs and it is advisable to carry out regular blood counts and urine analysis when patients take drugs over a long period of time.

Some nurses are allergic to some of these drugs. Gloves should be worn by those giving intramuscular injections and by anyone who is sensitive.

ANTI-DEPRESSANT DRUGS

Of the recently introduced drugs, some have a specifically anti-depressant effect. Some doctors use anti-depressant drugs in preference to electroconvulsive therapy. Some chronic depressive states have responded to drug treatment.

One group of these anti-depressant drugs (monoamine oxidiase inhibitors) can produce liver damage. They are also sometimes associated with severe headaches. Patients should not eat cheese or yeast extracts when they are taking these drugs and should avoid taking alcohol. Because it is dangerous to combine these drugs with certain other drugs, any change in prescription has to be preceded by a period when the patient is without any drugs.

Another group of anti-depressant drugs are collectively termed 'thymoleptic' drugs. There are fewer undesirable side effects but it takes up to 3 weeks before these drugs produce beneficial effects.

BOOKS FOR FURTHER READING

W. Sargent and E. Slater. (1963) *An Introduction to Physical Methods of Treatment in Psychiatry.* Livingstone, Edinburgh.

CHAPTER 23

Psychotherapy

The Purpose of Psychotherapy

Psychotherapy is considered to be the appropriate treatment when the patient's difficulties are thought to be caused by environmental influences of the past and his attitudes determined by factors in his early upbringing and childhood experiences.

Successful psychotherapy helps the patient to develop insight into his difficulties, to become aware of the chain of events which have led to his present condition and to gain some understanding of the motives of his behaviour.

Several forms of psychotherapy can be practised. The choice of specific method of psychotherapy depends on the patient's age. intelligence and degree of illness, and also on the psychiatrist's own training and attitude.

All psychotherapy is based on similar fundamental principles. In psychotherapy a relationship develops between therapist and patient, a relationship which helps the patient to resolve previously unrecognized conflicts and to achieve a better adaptation to stresses in life.

The process of psychotherapy is one in which the therapist listens with interest and attention to all the patient says and also notices the things the patient omits to say. The therapist's attitude, and his words, convey that it is safe for the patient, not only to talk, but also to allow his feelings free rein.

The patient needs to understand and accept that

psychological difficulties are as real as physical ones. He must recognize them to be just as serious as physical ones and must feel able to accept that, just like physical disorders, they require medical assistance to resolve them.

The patient, having gained confidence in the psychiatrist and established rapport in a preliminary interview, feels able to speak freely of anything that comes into his mind without fear of criticism or ridicule.

All psychotherapy consists of communication between the therapist and the patient. In the first few interviews the psychiatrist tends to be active in encouraging the patient to speak. He needs a detailed history; if necessary, and with the patient's permission, supplemented by information from relatives. During these early interviews the psychiatrist can gain a certain amount of understanding of the patient's problems. He cannot, at this stage, expect the patient to have developed much understanding but on the basis of his own understanding, the further course of action is planned.

The psychiatrist may decide on a course of intensive psychotherapy or he may decide to offer the patient supportive psychotherapy.

Intensive psychotherapy consists of many regular interviews—possibly 3 to 4 times per week for several years. The aim of such therapy is a fundamental restructuring of the patient's personality. The more disabling the patient's internal pressures the more he may feel in need of such complete reappraisal of his life. Intensive psychotherapy is anxiety producing and very slow to show tangible results. It is more likely to be successful if the patient's intelligence is relatively high. Because it is very time-consuming, for both the psychiatrist and the patient, it is a very expensive form of treatment. Irrespective of whether the patient bears the cost himself or whether the treatment is carried out under the National Health Service, the decision to embark on such a long term commitment has to be reached after very careful consideration of all the factors involved.

Supportive psychotherapy is a form of treatment in which the aim is the relief of symptoms and the reduction of stress. It is assumed that the healthy part of the patient's personality can reassert itself when the current crisis is resolved. Supportive psychotherapy does not aim at uncovering the patient's unconscious conflicts. On the contrary, it aims at achieving better developed defence mechanisms and greater self-confidence. Supportive psychotherapy focuses on the symptoms of which the patient complains and on the problems which beset him at the time of treatment. It does not necessarily require that the patient should gain insight into the casual connection between past experiences and present difficulties.

The decision about the form which psychotherapy is to take depends to a certain extent on the patient's own hopes and aims. It is only possible to treat a patient by psychotherapy if the patient himself makes that decision. Psychotherapy is not a form of treatment which the doctor actively administers and to which the patient passively submits. The patient in fact does all the active work of talking, thinking, reformulating and reappraising. The extent to which he is prepared to do so must determine the treatment objectives. Ultimately the patient must find his own solution and make his own decisions, though he does so with the help of the psychiatrist. It is important to know what kind of life the patient imagines for himself, with what kind of adaptation he would be satisfied, what kind of person he wants to be.

TECHNIQUES OF PSYCHOTHERAPY

The techniques of psychotherapy are based on the methods first developed by Freud, but a number of modifications have taken place.

Psychoanalysis, the technique used by Freud himself, was based on free association. The analyst gives no instructions whatever beyond the encouragement to say whatever comes to mind, however trivial or silly it may appear to the patient. As the latter continues to talk to the doctor he remembers more and more details of his past life, details of which he himself has been totally unaware. Each story brings to mind another one. Sometimes the patient finds it difficult to understand why a particular event has been recalled and how various ideas are connected.

Some events are recalled with considerable show of emotion which is often surprising to the patient. This emotional release, termed 'catharsis', is often experienced as a therapeutic event. As the story unfolds the doctor becomes aware of some of the mechanisms which were at work in making the patient the sort of person he is. He can observe what kind of statements are accompanied by deep emotion, such as grief or anger. He recognizes the patient's hostility to some of the people about whom he speaks, and his love for others. He picks out from the mass of recollections those facts which appear to have had a profound effect on the patient's subsequent development and begins to understand the patient's illness. It is not enough, though, that the doctor should understand the patient's illness, the patient himself must understand it.

Psychoanalysts will do nothing to speed up the process of developing insight. They wait patiently until the patient sees the connections between his present attitudes and his past experiences. Other psychiatrists make tentative interpretations to the patient which the latter may be able to accept as true. He may reject most vigorously interpretations which are nevertheless correct, only later to recognize their truth. He may accept the doctor's explanation but not really feel that he understands. Sometimes the patient's reactions show quite clearly that the doctor has been on the wrong track. Once the patient has begun to understand the reasons for his attitudes and his behaviour he may be able to attempt to modify them, and improvement may begin.

Psychiatrists who are not Freudian analysts tend to be more active in offering interpretations and in guiding patients towards discussion of topics which seem significant.

Hypnosis is used by some psychiatrists to assist the patient's recall of dramatic events or to make suggestions to the patient.

If the patient feels he would like to be able to talk but finds it hard to overcome his own resistance, drugs are at times used. Intravenous administration of such drugs as sodium amytal or pentothal or the administration of carbon dioxide often facilitate communication by the patient. Recall of painful events is often accompanied by extremely violent emotional experiences which the patient might find hard to tolerate without the help of drugs. Bringing into consciousness emotional difficulties which have been repressed is called 'abreaction'. The drug lysergic acid, usually referred to as L.S.D., has similar effects in producing emotional release. (It is one of the 'hallucinogens', a drug which produces hallucinatory experiences similar to those observed in some patients suffering from schizophrenia. This effect has stimulated research into schizophrenia.)

The root of the patient's trouble may be looked for in the very earliest childhood experiences, in the circumstances of birth, methods of feeding, weaning in babyhood, toilet training, in parental attitudes to the patient as an infant, and the small child's attitude to his siblings.

During intensive psychotherapy the patient may be able to recall feelings of these earliest periods of life. There are times when the patient not only remembers, but effectively re-lives these early experiences. His behaviour 'regresses' to a very early stage of development.

The psychiatrist's passive role in psychotherapy is often imperfectly understood. In the early stages of treatment patients may feel disappointed because the psychiatrist does not make positive suggestions or give positive advice. Most psychiatrists refrain from giving any advice, because such action would take away from the patient responsibility for his behaviour. There are some patients, however, for whom a more positive approach appears indicated. Suggestion and reassurance may then play a part in psychotherapy. The psychiatrist's manner, impressiveness and air of competence may play a part in suggesting that the patient is in good hands and the psychiatrist's utterances can help to suggest that the patient is capable of constructive behaviour and of finding a solution to his problems. Reassurance may deal with specific fears, for example a fear that the patient is becoming insane or that his symptoms are unique and beyond the doctor's understanding.

Occasionally positive, didactic teaching about matters of health, for example, about the physiological concomitants of anxiety, may accompany psychotherapy.

During psychotherapy, whatever form it may take, there are periods of intense anxiety, when the patient finds it difficult to persevere with treatment. He is helped, during such phases, by the relationship he has formed with the psychiatrist. This relationship is partly determined by the psychiatrist's personality. Partly it is the kind of relationship which the patient, in the past, had with his parents, or with other significant people. The patient is said to have a 'transference' relationship with his psychiatrist. All the elements of love and hate of earlier relationships are repeated as 'positive or negative transference' for the psychiatrist. In his turn the psychiatrist often responds with feelings of resentment to hostility or with feelings of pleasure when the patient seems to be progressing. The psychiatrist's response to the patient is described as 'counter transference'.

Transference relationships are an important aid to the understanding of the patient's feelings and an important prop for the patient in turbulent periods of treatment.

Transference situations have to be resolved, however, before the patient can give up his dependence on the psychiatrist and decide to terminate treatment.

Most commonly patients receive psychotherapy either in out-patient clinics or privately. As psychotherapy progresses the patient's attitudes gradually change. New relationships develop, old ones undergo considerable modifications. New problems arise as the patient attempts to deal with situations which he has previously found difficult. As new problems arise the patient brings these to the psychiatrist and they form the starting point in the treatment session.

Only rarely does the patient require in-patient treatment during psychotherapy. The reason for admission to hospital may be severe disturbances caused by the treatment and the patient's relatives may find it impossible to give him the support he requires. Consequently patients who receive psychotherapy in hospital may be among those who are most difficult to nurse.

THE NURSE'S ROLE IN PSYCHOTHERAPY

Supportive Psychotherapy

The nurse fulfils various functions depending on the technique employed and on her understanding of the fundamental principles involved. Some psychiatrists are more willing than others to use nursing staff in psychotherapy. If the patient is receiving supportive psychotherapy the nurse's function is to manipulate the environment in such a way that the patient meets with fewer difficulties than he would outside the hospital.

She can reduce the demands made upon him and exert her influence in such a manner that he experiences his surroundings as being friendly, accepting and non-critical. In some instances, without modifying her behaviour in any way and without even a clear understanding of what is taking place, the nurse may be used by the patient to fulfil some of his needs. A patient who is insecure and dependent may lean on a forceful, confident nurse, deriving support and security. A patient who requires someone who is dependent on him may satisfy his need to be protective by trying to help a new nurse.

During the course of psychotherapy the nurse acts as a suitable person on whom to practise newly acquired social skills. She can serve as a target for the patient's emotions and because she remains unaffected and detached can help him to learn control over the expression of his feelings. With more understanding and greater skill the nurse can exploit her special relationship with the patient. She can do this either by her endeavour to minimize tension between therapeutic sessions, thus enabling the patient to use the interviews with the psychiatrist to better advantage, or in some instances she can help to extend the therapeutic sessions. The patient can talk to the nurse, using her to sort out some of his complicated thoughts, ideas and feelings, so making it easier for him to select the most important facts for the therapeutic interview with the doctor.

In some forms of psychotherapy the nurse assumes the role of a significant figure in the patient's life, and enables him to act out in the hospital setting the emotional responses usually triggered off by his own environment.

Psychotherapy always produces changes in the patient's attitude to other people. Different patients' reactions to each other, the way in which groups form and break up, the emergence of friendships and the development of love and hate reactions among patients are always significant as an indication of progress and as a stimulus to therapy. The nurse is in the best position to observe the ward as a whole, to assess the forces of which the ward group is composed, and to exert some influence on the climate of the ward in order to create a therapeutic community.

Role Therapy

Interpersonal relationships are of the utmost importance in all forms of psychotherapy. In supportive psychotherapy the patient casts the nurse into various roles, depending on his own previous relationships to other people. Role therapy is a form of treatment in which the nurses, under the guidance of the psychiatrist, deliberately try to assume a particular role-relationship towards the patient.

One of the nurses, for example, may deliberately behave towards the patient in the manner in which his father may have behaved and a re-enaction of the patient's attitude and behaviour towards the father is thus deliberately provoked. In this form of treatment it may be necessary to pool a great deal of information about the patient in order to plan the part which the doctor wishes one of the nurses to play. From time to time discussion between the members of the staff must take place.

If the patient finds it difficult to explain to the psychiatrist where his problems lie, if he lacks the intelligence or fluency to verbalize his difficulties, this method of treatment is often successful in recreating the problems before the doctor's very eyes. The psychiatrist need not rely on the patient's memory of past events, he can use current troubles as they arise to help the patient. As a result of the emotionally charged relationship which the patient develops towards the nurse concerned, the ward routine and hospital life produce the kind of reaction which may have led to the patient's admission. While, normally, mental hospital treatment owes its success to the avoidance of such scenes, in this form of therapy the repetition is deliberately created.

The patient can be helped in one of two ways. Attitudes and the approach of the nurses can help the patient to develop more adequate methods of solving his difficulties or, alternatively, the psychiatrist who is not in any way involved, utilizes the patient's trust in him to support him during each difficult phase. The doctor himself may adopt a role which is opposite to that adopted by the nurse and as a result of this he is felt to be on the patient's side. The patient feels able to give free rein to his feelings, to discuss and modify his attitudes and develop new ways of dealing with old problems, because he has the support of the doctor. The nurse, in a similar way to the patient's relatives before, partly causes the patient's disturbed behaviour and at the same time must find some method of dealing with each disturbance as it arises. The nurse has the advantage of previous experience and of relative emotional detachment. In spite of this she may find it difficult to maintain the one-sided relationship which is required in the situation, the patient being deeply attached or violently antagonistic to her, while she remains emotionally detached. She must deliberately act as if she were affected by the patient's emotional attitude, without, in fact, becoming emotionally so involved that she loses the ability to make sound judgements.

In order to maintain this relationship the nurse must have the help of her colleagues, with whom she must frequently discuss the patient, and her own attitude to him. Her colleagues may be able to point out any gestures or actions which may have indicated impatience or anger without her being aware of it. Discussion with her colleagues may also prevent undue friction among the nurses over the treatment of the patient. Quite frequently a patient who feels angry with one of the nurses ingratiates himself with another and tries to engage one nurse as an ally against another.

It may be most valuable to create the special role of an ally. Often the psychiatrist assumes this role in order to help the patient in his relationship with the nurse. It should be clearly understood by all concerned that somebody must accept the part of always being on the patient's side. But the situation should be planned by the psychiatrist, not created and exploited by the patient. If the latter succeeds in creating mistrust and mutual hostility among the nurses he will become frightened, and lose confidence in the hospital's power to help.

Deep Psychotherapy

The nurse's function if the patient is undergoing deep psychotherapy is similar in many ways. There is no need to adopt any particular role, and no need to fear that wrong approach could harm the patient. It is part of any form of deep psychotherapy that the patient is prepared to tell the therapist all his thoughts, which of course include any thoughts the patient may have about the nurses. It follows that the therapist is very well informed about the nurses' attitudes, their behaviour and the effect they have on the patient.

The therapist in turn has agreed to listen to the patient's comments, and to regard as confidential anything he may hear. He cannot divulge very much information to the nurses and may only very indirectly influence their attitudes to the patient.

This situation could be exceptionally difficult for nurses, who may feel that the patient is carrying tales to the doctor and that they are being criticized. Sometimes the patient's version of any incident which may have occurred in the ward may appear exaggerated to the nurse and she may feel hurt and insulted if she thinks that the patient's story is believed and that she is not even given a chance to explain.

Nurses should try to understand that this one-sided relationship is fundamental to psychotherapy.

If the patient is treated as an out-patient he may for instance complain that his wife rejects him. This may not be a true statement of fact. The wife may not really reject him at all and may tell about the husband's coldness to her with as much conviction as the husband showed in his version. It does not really matter who is right. If the husband is the patient, his way of experiencing the situation is all-important. The wife, too, may need help and usually the social worker will offer it to her.

If the patient is an in-patient the relationship to the nurse is parallel to the one described. It does not matter in the least whether the patient's story is true, all that matters is how it appears to the patient. Nurses may require some help in the same way as the patient's relatives, but usually they can give each other the necessary support.

During deep psychotherapy the patient may pass through a series of extremely difficult phases. He may become acutely depressed, and require careful supervision if there is any risk of suicide. In this case the psychiatrist usually warns the nurses, although this is contrary to the usual practice in psychotherapy.

Periods of excitement, of aggressive behaviour, of violent emotional outbursts, are more difficult to predict and the nurses must manage to the best of their ability to help the patient through the difficult phase. Often these disturbances follow significant interviews, or take place when a particularly painful interview is approaching.

The patient dreams more vividly as he acquires practice in relating his dreams, and often a disturbed night is followed by a day of irritability and moodiness. Sometimes it appears as if treatment is making the patient worse. This is deceptive. Often real improvement follows when the patient has successfully worked through a particularly painful period of his life. At times the patient himself feels despondent about his treatment and this may reinforce the nurses' belief that psychotherapy is not helping very much.

At certain phases of treatment the patient shows a marked resistance to therapy. He forgets his appointments, finds excuses for not attending and is apt to belittle the effect of treatment in his conversation with the nurses. The latter should not fail to understand that the patient's resistance is an indication that a crucial point in treatment is being reached. Discontinuation of treatment may well occur if they reinforce the patient's sceptical attitude.

GROUP THERAPY

Group therapy is a form of psychotherapy which is time saving, because by these means many problems common to several patients can be cleared up jointly. The therapist is able to give more time to the group of patients than he could separately to each individual.

Many patients are helped by group therapy in a more specific way. Diffidence is gradually overcome by listening to other patients discussing their difficulties, and it is possible slowly to gain the courage necessary to speak about personal problems. Listening to others makes the patient realize that he is not alone in his troubles, and that his difficulties are not unique. Often the patient believes that he would be rejected if more were known about his personality. To hear others relate similar facts about themselves without losing sympathy or acceptance may be beneficial.

It is often easier for an individual to understand the mechanism underlying other people's neurotic symptoms than to gain insight into the causation of his own behaviour. A growing awareness of his own motivation may be possible for him as a member of a group.

Group therapy may take place by appointment on an

out-patient basis, or may form part of the treatment programme during in-patient therapy.

Group psychotherapy has many of the characteristic features of individual psychotherapy. As a form of intensive psychotherapy a group of 6 to 8 members usually meet regularly with the analyst whose attitude to the group as a whole corresponds to that of the analyst in individual treatment. Therapeutic groups of this nature are usually 'closed' groups, i.e. all patients start and terminate treatment simultaneously. No new members are admitted. It is difficult for such groups to deal with observers, and consequently nurses are not usually present during therapeutic sessions.

Conflicts with which the group deals are related to group membership as well as to the specific problems of individual members. Patients spend only a short period of their day in group sessions. Any anxiety which remains unresolved is taken back to the ward group as a whole and affects the total management of the ward.

Group therapy can also follow the pattern of supportive psychotherapy. Groups of patients meet regularly discussing, in the first instance, any topic of current interest to the ward. Such groups are usually 'open' groups. New patients can be invited to join and as patients recover they leave the group. In group therapy of this kind one staff member assumes the role of convener of the group. Often this is a psychiatrist but, increasingly, nurses are developing skills in the management of such therapeutic groups.

In group therapy of this kind it is possible and desirable to have observers, who are able to note and report the various forces which act in the group. The presence of an observer is of course one of the factors which influence what happens.

In therapeutic groups of this kind the events of the ward often form the official part of the agenda. The way patients organize their time, the manner in which they carry out their responsibility, the frustrations they experience in relation to the hospital staff are profitable topics for discussion. They constitute common business and, therefore, offer an opportunity to all to contribute to the discussion. The way patients use this opportunity reflects their personal problems and attitudes. Some patients find it very difficult to speak, and it is the business of the other members of the group to explore the reasons for the difficulty and to help the patient to deal with it. Patients who monopolise the floor during a meeting similarly give others the opportunity to understand their need to dominate and to deal with the situation.

There are often long silences during group meetings, when the leader waits for tensions to become manifest or for topics of high priority to emerge. Facile chatter about trivialities often occurs when some important business threatens to be too painful to discuss. Chatter is pleasant for the group members. Silence is difficult to tolerate; yet silence can be a very important part of treatment. During a period of silence members can examine their feelings towards each other and towards the therapist. They become aware of hostility and tensions or of depressive moods or thoughtful reflection. During a period of silence people often watch each other and detect signs of anxiety by the way people fidget or pass around cigarettes, or tap their feet, or hide their faces. During a period of silence they can also sometimes detect genuine interest or concern or sympathy in the faces of other patients or of staff members. Knowing when and how to break a silence is very difficult. If it has gone on too long it becomes very difficult to break but if the leader is anxious about silence he may deprive some members of the group of valuable experience.

In many group meetings patients express criticism of the staff.

This is to be encouraged for a number of reasons. Patients need a safe outlet for their hostile feelings. At some stage staff are certain to become targets of such feelings. Group meetings should provide a safe forum for discussion and in this way help the patient to cope. The patient's feelings may in the course of such discussion become more obvious to the staff and to other patients, who as a result of this may understand the problem better and become more able to help.

The patients may gain insight into their own problems as a result of the response they obtain from members of the group.

Of course it is always possible that good grounds exist for patients' complaints about the staff. Patients' complaints should not automatically be regarded as evidence of displaced feeling.

There is a danger that a split may occur between patients and staff if the staff react defensively to the patients' complaints. To be effective, groups need to develop a certain cohesion and identity. If staff members predominate in number or in articulateness, two groups tend to form instead of one, a staff and a patient group, with rivalry and competition instead of co-operative effort.

During group meetings a certain amount of clarification takes place of the patients' problems. By making observations about the patients' behaviour, rewording certain statements, explaining how the problem appears to the onlooker and tentatively interpreting what it might mean, patients begin to gain a new level of understanding of their own and other patients' difficulties. One of the advantages of group therapy lies in the fact that patients can exert therapeutic influences on each other.

This will be discussed more fully in Chapter 27.

CHAPTER 24

Behaviour Therapy

MALADAPTIVE behaviour is generally recognized to have its origin earlier in life. Psychotherapy is based on the assumption that *insight* into connections between earlier experience and current difficulties is therapeutic. It is sometimes possible to bring about changes in behaviour more easily by assuming that the maladaptive behaviour is learned and that new and better adaptive behaviour can also be *learned*.

Behaviour therapy makes use of the knowledge derived from the psychology of learning. It is most effective when the aim of treatment is to change isolated aspects of behaviour rather than the patient's total response pattern.

Isolated habits—for example, nailbiting—or isolated phobias—for example, the fear of boarding a bus—or single symptoms such as bedwetting can be treated successfully by behaviour therapy.

Aversion treatment used in the treatment of alcoholism is one form of behaviour therapy.

The most important factor in learning is 'reinforcement'. Whenever any particular form of behaviour is rewarded it is more likely to be repeated than behaviour which is unrewarded. Children learn how to behave either because they receive some tangible rewards such as sweets when successful, or because mother's approval and love act as reward for certain forms of behaviour, but are withheld for other forms of behaviour. Reward acts as reinforcement.

Sometimes maladaptive behaviour is accidentally rewarded. A child who cries may attract its mother's love and protection and learn to cry in order to obtain affection and protection. Later in life crying turns out to be maladaptive; it no longer attracts the reward of early childhood days but by then the response of crying may be so firmly established that it is used in spite of being maladaptive.

Such symptoms as phobias of open spaces originally bring the reward of protection from danger. They continue later even though their disadvantages may far outweigh the positive reward they attract.

At times there is a small immediate gain to be derived from neurotic symptoms and this reinforces the maladaptive pattern of behaviour, though in the long run no gain ensues.

When an attempt is made to unlearn a habit pattern which is firmly established a number of procedures can be adopted:

Operant Conditioning

In this form of treatment an opportunity is created to reinforce the appropriate behaviour and every attempt is made to avoid maladaptive behaviour occurring.

In the treatment of neurotic children, for example, various methods are used to wake the child before it wets the bed. Whenever it wakes in a dry bed it is rewarded. Finding ways of lightening the child's sleep and of rousing it as the bladder becomes full, or as the first drops of urine are passed, helps increase the likelihood of a dry night occurring again.

Attempts have been made to treat stammering by the method of operant conditioning. Some research is being carried out in the treatment of childhood autism. It is argued that the usual practice in treatment is to give love to the child when it appears to be withdrawn. This reinforces withdrawal. Instead it is suggested that reinforcing those occasions when the child makes an approach to a person, or an attempt to communicate, might be a more effective treatment.

Reciprocal Inhibition

A form of treatment in which those responses are rewarded which are the opposite to the anxiety responses one wishes to eliminate.

Many patients suffer from anxiety in relation to a number of situations—not only boarding a bus, for example, may arouse anxiety, but also boarding a taxi, though maybe to a lesser extent, and travelling in a private car, though perhaps least. The treatment consists of listing all those situations in which the patient feels anxious, arranging these situations in order, from the most to the least anxiety-provoking.

The patient is then helped to relax by the use of hypnotic drugs or hypnosis, and in this condition, invited to imagine the situation lowest in order of anxiety rating. To be able to do so without anxiety acts as an inhibiting factor and anxiety is gradually unlearnt. If successful with the least disturbing stimulus the patient goes on to the stimulus situation next on the list in the order of seriousness. Three or four situations are visualized in each treatment session. When the patient can imagine the situation without anxiety it is easier to expose himself to the real life situation, and success then reinforces learning.

With both operant conditioning and reciprocal inhibition it is important that real life stresses should not interfere with the orderly progress of behaviour therapy. The exposure to anxiety-provoking stimuli is carefully graduated during treatment. It would be harmful if the requirements of the ward routine were to force the patient prematurely to expose himself to the stresses of the most anxiety provoking situation.

A patient in a phobic state can, for example, by

behaviour therapy, be gradually helped to leave his bedroom, then the ward, then risk entering the common room, then the dining room, then perhaps the entertainment hall before being expected to leave the hospital to go to a place of public entertainment. If a patient who is still trying to cope with the dining room were forced to go with the other patients to a theatre in town there could be a serious setback in his treatment.

The nurse's function in behaviour therapy often consists of protecting the patient from demands made on him by the ward community. This may mean that special rules may have to be made for such patients. This of course raises the possibility, either, that nonconforming is being rewarded and reinforced, or that the other patients' jealousy and hostility create new anxieties, which counterbalance the benefit gained from treatment.

Aversion Threapy

A form of behaviour therapy in which the process of 'deconditioning' is used. Patients suffering from alcoholism are treated by aversion therapy. The aim is to destroy the association between drinking and pleasure, by substituting for it a conditioned response of aversion to alcohol.

The patient, on several occasions, is given an emetic with his drink. The feeling of nausea which results from the emetic will gradually become a conditioned response to drinking alcohol, to the smell of alcohol or even the thought of drinking alcohol.

Although this method of establishing a conditioned response of nausea to alcohol is often effective, the results are not lasting unless the connection between vomiting and alcohol is periodically repeated by the use of an emetic.

The use of Antabuse helps the patient to maintain the conditioned response, because every time the patient takes a drink he experiences again the unpleasant effects of the interaction of antebuse and alcohol. The aversion to alcohol is thus reinforced.

Aversion therapy has also been used for patients suffering from sexual perversions.

Patients undergoing aversion therapy require the support of a sympathic and optimistic person. It is often difficult for the patient to feel in any way positive about the treatment. The unpleasantness is so great that there are many occasions when the patient does not feel it worth while to continue. His despondency may take on suicidal proportions.

The symptoms which are removed by behaviour therapy may at first sight appear to be isolated and the patient may otherwise have appeared healthy and well adjusted. When the symptoms disappear the full impact of the patient's underlying disorder may become evident, and more intensive therapy may become necessary. This is particularly the case with patients suffering from alcoholism or from sexual perversion whose whole social life may have been determined by their disorder. When such patients sever their association with fellow sufferers their underlying personality problems may become evident.

CHAPTER 25

Nurse – Patient Relationships

IT was said earlier that the progress of psychotherapy depends on the relationship which develops between the therapist and the patient.

The relationship between the doctor and the patient in psychotherapy is unique, and it is based on the understanding that communications between the patient and his doctor are absolutely confidential. Nurses are therefore often ignorant of what goes on in psychotherapy sessions.

The patient may feel somewhat suspicious of the staff, wondering if the promise of confidentiality is being kept. His conversation with the nurses may be designed to test whether the trust in the doctor is well founded. It is in such a case helpful to the patient, to find that nurses do not have access to case notes and only know as much about him as he himself chooses to disclose to the nurse. The patient may also derive comfort from observing the fact that case notes are carefully locked away.

To the nursing staff communication about the patient is important if they are to act intelligently and as a team. In the case of patients undergoing psychotherapy such communication is however best carried out in verbal reporting and in staff meetings rather than by reading case notes which contain confidential information. In the first instance, at any rate, it is easier for the nurse to approach the patient if she is unbiased and uninfluenced by advance information.

In some hospitals it is the practice to keep full psycho-therapy notes locked away, but to make available to the staff notes in form of a summary, so that some degree of planning is possible.

Often the relationship between doctor and patient is not the only significant relationship to occur during the patient's stay in hospital. Other members of staff may develop relationships with the patient, which have therapeutic or anti-therapeutic results. By design or by accident members of staff other than the patient's doctor may even take on the main therapeutic role.

The term relationship is one which is employed differently by different people. Nurses sometimes use adjectives like 'good' or 'bad' to qualify the word relationship, when they discuss what happens between the patient and themselves. Such judgements are often invalid, as it is extremely difficult to describe what kind of relationship is good or bad for the patient. It may be good for the patient to have a negative relationship, for example one of hostility towards a nurse, if this enables the patient to discuss his feelings, not only about the nurse but about other significant people in his life. It may be bad for the patient to have a positive relationship with a nurse, if such a relationship allows the patient to remain excessively dependent, or if it prevents explora-tion of aggressive feelings.

The pattern of relationships into which any person enters changes throughout life. Every contact a person makes contributes something towards the formation of relationships and the quality of every human contact depends to some extent on the relationships which already exist. Without contact with people one cannot learn to relate to them. A child who has very little contact with its mother for example cannot learn to enter into a relationship with her. Only repeated con-tact with the mother enables the child to develop trust and love, and only repeated contact with the child enables the mother to develop the concern and tenderness for the child which are characteristic of a mother–child relationship. When a mother–child relationship has been established, its existence affects every contact the mother and child have with each other. The mother's correction is acceptable to the child or the child's temper is acceptable to the mother because of the relationship which already exists between them. The child allows and expects the mother to bathe it, tuck it up in bed and kiss it, activities which it would resent from a stranger with whom it has no loving relationship.

Relationships between people are always characterized by their emotional content. Loving, caring for, prizing, being concerned, are the positive emotional characteristics; hating, feeling angry, disappointed or frustrated, the negative emotional characteristics of relationships between people. Loving and hating often occur together; being pleased and disappointed are the opposite sides of the same coin in a relationship. One cannot feel angry with a person about whom one does not care, one cannot hate a person whom one does not also, at other times, love.

In the course of life one establishes relationships with people differing in quality, in intensity and in the extent to which they are reciprocated.

The relationships between mother and child or between father and child or between siblings often develop into the prototypes of the kind of relationships one enters into later in life. Mother–child relationships and father–child relationships are different in quality but may be similiar in intensity.

In any relationship between two people, the participants may have similar or dissimilar status, and their roles in relation to each other may be alike or different. The parents' role differs from that of the children. Parents are expected to give care, children to receive care; parents are expected to be protective, children are expected to be dependent. The parents' status is different from that of their children. Status determines the rights and obligations of each participant in a relationship. The parents' status entitles them to give commands and administer punishment. The children's status obliges them to obey and to submit but gives them the right to behave in childish irresponsible ways. As children grow up role and status change in the parent–child relationship often accompanied by a considerable amount of conflict.

Sibling relationships and friendships are relationships in which the participants' roles are similar and status is equal.

The way in which people address each other is often an indication of the extent to which reciprocity exists in the relationship. Children address their parents as 'mother', or 'dad', parents call their children by Christian names, or sometimes nicknames. Friends, or brother and sister, call each other by Christian names.

Many patients have experienced, in childhood, difficulties in some of their basic relationships. These difficulties have resulted in disturbed relationships with people in adult life. Marital problems, difficulties in coping with employers, problems in dealing with subordinates are often indications that the patient has failed to come to terms with his own changing role and status in society. Experience of life in hospital should enable the patient to learn how to deal more effectively with the changing relationships into which he enters.

The very fact that a person has decided to become a patient allocates to him a special role and a new status. It becomes the role of a patient to be dependent, trusting, submissive, and rather like a child. A patient has a special status in being the most important person in the hospital, the person whose existence justifies the existence of the whole organization. On the other hand,

the patient's status is low. He cannot exercise his right
to make decisions and has abdicated from responsibility.

The role and status of a patient is in fact very similar
to that of a child. The patient's need for protection
causes him to cast members of staff into parental roles.
He assigns to the staff superior status, and expects from
them behaviour appropriate to that of father or mother.

The parental role is one which the nurse often
assumes; often with beneficial results, but accompanied
by certain disadvantages. It may be appropriate to
examine in detail what is involved when a nurse takes on
a mothering role. It entails authority on the part of the
nurse and submission on the part of the patient. The
nurse takes on certain commitments to the patient. It is
a one-sided relationship. The nurse is concerned with
the patient's welfare, not her own, with the patient's
thoughts, feelings, interests and problems, not with her
own. In her mothering role she has to be accepting of
the patient, no matter what his behaviour may be. Her
acceptance is unconditional. Yet it is also her duty in her
mothering role to indicate disapproval and disappointment. As a mother, she gives encouragement and support,
always expecting the capacity to improve and to excel,
yet knowing and making allowances for shortcomings.

In her mothering role the nurse is not only concerned
with the patient while he is in her physical presence.
She is concerned with all he does. She knows his friends
and their influence on him. She is interested in what he
learns and how he spends his leisure. She arranges for
him to be looked after by others when she is not available
herself, or when she cannot help. When the patient is in
need of a dentist for example, she arranges it, accompanies the patient and afterwards is concerned with
comforting him if he is in pain. She is concerned also
with aspirations and plans for the future.

The mothering role can provide considerable satisfaction to the nurse and to the patient, so much so that the patient may be prevented from outgrowing his dependency. Good mothering makes provision for growing independence, but the authoritarian attitude of some nurses makes it difficult for them to recognize this.

The mothering role of the nurse and the function of a real mother are dissimilar in many ways. In real life the role of the mother is complementary to that of the father. Conflicts between father and mother about the child, and jealousies between children about their parents are normal events in family relationships. Father and mother have an important relationship with each other, which is significant to the children.

In hospital it is almost impossible for such triangular relationships to be reproduced. Often the nurse may have to assume the role of father and mother—of authority and protection simultaneously, making it difficult for her to be as accepting as she might like to be.

When a doctor or another nurse take on the father role, difficulties may arise in the sharing of parental functions. Relationships between the nurse and the doctor can never be as close as is expected of father and mother. It is argued, however, that the special kind of love–hate relationship which sometimes exists between doctor and ward sister is the result of the rivalry situation into which patients cast them.

Relationships between doctor and nurse are seldom close enough to withstand serious disagreement about a patient, and the resulting anxiety tends to spread rapidly from the nursing staff to the patients. Because the patient's anxiety appears to aggravate rather than improve his condition, the beneficial effects of the relationship with the nurse are often obscured.

Relationships often get strained when they are exposed to public scrutiny and criticism. Nurses' relationships with their patients are often scrutinized by others, higher in the nursing hierarchy. Any indication that the patient's behaviour meets with disapproval may make the nurse feel defensive and inadequate in her role performance.

The greatest difficulties in fulfilling a mothering role towards a patient are related to the staffing pattern of the wards and the nurse's responsibility to a number of patients. In real life only one person has the role of mother. Even if mother is asleep, or ill, or away, her place cannot be filled by anyone else; attempts by paid helpers or by grandparents to substitute can never be wholly successful while a real mother exists. In hospital the nurse's mothering role is confined to her hours of duty. When she is on holiday or ill or off duty someone else automatically steps in. Real mothering only comes to an abrupt end through death. The hospital relationship between the nurse and the patient comes to an end when the nurse decides to leave, or when she is moved to another ward. Even when a patient is very well prepared for the separation resentment and grief are inevitable, if the relationship had any emotional significance for the patient. The more the relationship between the patient and nurse resembled a mother–child relationship, the more damaging sudden termination of the relationship will be.

If a patient whose relationship with his own mother was unsatisfactory is to gain any benefit from experiencing a mothering relationship with a nurse, his new experience should be a corrective one, not one that reinforces his expectation of disappointment and frustration.

Because the hospital organization is such that the patient is almost certain to be disappointed, it would seem that something other than spontaneous mothering activity is required from the nurse.

Nurses and patients sometimes enter into relationships which resemble sibling relationships or friendships more than mother–child relationships. If the nurse can fulfil the role of friend or older brother or sister, the patient may benefit by using her as a model on which to pattern his own behaviour, or by indentifying with her and consequently becoming aware of his own positive attributes.

Many patients need friends. Their isolation from people and inability to make and keep friends may be the cause or the result of their illness. The opportunity to find a friend in hospital may be of great therapeutic significance. The relationship between the nurse and the patient cannot, however, develop into real friendship. What characterizes friendship or sibling relationships is mutual trust and mutual exchange of confidence. Friends make demands on each other and take it for granted that their demands will be met. Friends treat each other as equals, share each other's troubles and difficulties. It is not possible for the nurse to burden the patient with her problems or with her personal affairs, and consequently, the relationship becomes one-sided. The choice of meeting places and the duration of contacts is often one-sidedly determined to suit the convenience of the nurse not the patient. In conversation between the nurse and the patient the focus is on the need of the patient, not the need of the nurse. The relationship between nurse and patient is often of greater importance to the patient than it is to the nurse. To the patient it may seem a unique relationship—the nurse may be the only or the best friend the patient ever had. But to the nurse the patient is only one of many with whom she relates. Her personal family or friends provide the satisfaction of closer bonds. She does not regard her relationship with the patient as a significant event in her own life and she does not plan that the 'relationship should continue indefinitely. If the patient regards the relationship with the nurse as a personal, rather than a professional one he may become disappointed and his previous anti-social attitudes may be reinforced.

There are occasions when the nurse does put herself in the role of friend to the patient, and the actions of a friend come to be expected by the patient. This may occur because of an intuitive affinity between the two people concerned. More often it occurs because the patient's suffering is particularly obvious and his appeals for help particularly urgent. The patient may succeed in making the nurse feel sure that she understands him much better than anyone else, and that only she can be relied on to provide the right approach and the right support. This kind of relationship is rarely beneficial to the patient. It leads to increasing demands and as the nurse begins to feel resentful of these demands, she tends to withdraw her support. The fact that the patient is not responding causes the nurse to feel guilty and disappointed and eventually angry with the patient.

The nurse who feels that she has some special ability to help the patient, which others lack, tends to be criticized and resented by her colleagues.

The term 'involvement' is sometimes used to describe this relationship in which the nurse's own emotions render her unable to view the patient's problems objectively, and in which the patient's lack of progress becomes a personal challenge to the nurse. Nurses tend to become secretive about such relationships. The patient in the long run tends to be let down and the nurse to become profoundly unhappy.

It is possible to prevent relationships between the nurse and the patient from reaching an untherapeutic level, by ensuring that free discussion takes place between nurses about their feelings for the patients, and their feelings about each other. To expose one's work to the critical evaluation of one's colleagues is not easy, but it is a necessary corrective and support.

To become emotionally involved may not be helpful to the patient, but it cannot be prevented by prohibitions or warnings of danger. The secrecy often surrounding involvement may be the result of expected disapproval. Instead of pretending that involvement does not occur, it is better to acknowledge its existence and co-operate with colleagues in finding a solution to the problem.

A solution may be found by trying to establish a transference relationship rather than one of personal friendship. In a transference relationship the patient uses the nurse in place of his own friends or relations to become the target for love and hate, and the object of admiration and criticism. The termination of such a relationship is carefully planned as a part of the treatment.

A transference relationship is similar to the relationship which the patient forms with a psychotherapist. Such relationships enable the patient to experience close human contact, to enjoy approval and encouragement without the danger of being disappointed. They help the patient to face his feelings and to cope with them.

It is essential that the nurse should be capable of deep feeling for and emotional understanding of the patient, and that she should have insight into her own emotional response to the patient. One way to achieve such insight would be for each nurse to undergo a personal analysis; but few people would consider this practicable or desirable. Some people advocate instead a systematic review of what goes on between the nurse and a patient; by a process of regular supervision from a trained person. This method is adopted in the training for social case work. Regular group discussion with the members of the ward team in an atmosphere of acceptance and co-operation may be the most effective way of alerting nurses to the significance of their own attitude and behaviour.

CHAPTER 26

Nurse – Patient Interactions

DURING his stay in hospital the patient establishes contact with many people. His contacts with other patients may be the most helpful and significant ones. These will be discussed in the next chapter. Here the contacts with nurses are discussed.

During the first few days in hospital the patient is among strangers. He naturally feels insecure and diffident. His attitude to the people who are concerned with his treatment is affected by this. Some people show their anxiety, others appear full of self-confidence or even a little brash or aggressive. When the patient settles, his behaviour may be very different from the initial impression he created. It is important to take his first approach seriously, as his attitude on admission may be characteristic of the way in which he behaves towards strangers. His shyness and diffidence or his apparent aggressiveness may be part of his difficulty in meeting people.

The preliminary period of getting to know one another is a very important phase in establishing confidence. No patient is quite free from preconceived ideas. 'Hospital', 'psychiatric hospital', 'nurse', 'psychiatric patient', are all words which conjure up mental pictures for everybody, pictures which often correspond very little to reality and are determined by past experience and by some ideal which is popularly accepted.

The patient's ready-made attitude to nurses may be important in helping him to accept hospitalization. To many people the title 'nurse' and the nurse's uniform stand for all that is good, kind and competent. This stereotype is, of course, quite unrealistic; nurses are people, each nurse is different and no nurse embodies all the good qualities which patients expect in the ideal nurse. Nevertheless, the fact that patients tend to be well disposed to nurses and to trust them may reduce their anxiety on admission.

The presence of nurses may also help to convince the suspicious patient that he really is in hospital and to accept that he is ill. This first, reassuring effect of the nurse's uniform may possibly be the only justification for wearing a uniform at all. The wearing of uniform becomes harmful if it gives the nurse a false sense of security and leads her to adopt an attitude of authority and superiority over the patients, which is incompatible with a thera-peutic attitude. Uniform has the effect of giving to all who wear it, similar roles and status. When a patient needs a nurse, any one of the people in a nurse's uniform will satisfy his needs, but by the end of the first few days a patient in a psychiatric ward knows each nurse as an individual and has formed an opinion of each.

If nurses did not wear uniform they might find it easier to accept the fact that they must establish 'their position' in the ward personally and cannot expect to be treated with respect as of right.

Introductions are important in stressing the nurse's personality rather than her role. The patient is often more interested in her name than in her rank in the nursing hierarchy. Many patients appreciate it if nurses are willing to be called by Christian names.

The process of becoming acquainted is a mutual one. While the nurse tries to find out as much as she can about the patient in order to help him, the patient tries to find out as much as he can about the nurses in order to establish which ones can be trusted. Some patients try to ask questions about personal matters and attempt to interview the nurse about her family, her social life, her views and interests. There is no need to answer such questions. They can be deflected by indicating that the nurse is more interested in talking about the patient than about herself.

The nurse gets to know the patient in conversation and in joint activities. Some nurses find it easier to contact the patient while some activity is in progress. The personal attention which the nurse gives to the patient gives the opportunity for communication. The nurse who admits the patient, who deals with his property and clothing, who shows the patient around the ward and who has met and spoken to the relatives on the first day is often the one in whom the patient feels particularly confident. If the patient requires help with bathing or personal hygiene, if the nurse assists in keeping the patient's clothes washed and ironed or if she takes a particular interest in the patient's hair style or grooming she may become especially acceptable. The daily round of ward cleaning and preparation for meals are good points of contact.

Everything the patient does in the hospital should be fully shared by nurses. The patient's work in the occupation department, his activities at entertainments, his use of leisure in the ward, should be of interest to the nurse both at the time when the nurse is present and participates, and later as topics of conversation. The more common experience the nurse has with the patient, the easier she will find it to talk to him. The fact that the nurse shows interest in the patient's daily life encourages him to believe that she has his interest at heart.

Conversation with the patient rarely touches on personal problems in the early stages. At no time should the nurse ask direct questions or appear to be prying. The aim of talking to the patient is not to find out about his illness, but to get to know him as a person. Anything that interests the patient is a good starting point—clothes, sports, the patient's occupation, the radio or television programme, the contents of the newspaper. Gradually it becomes possible to build up a picture of the way the patient spent his life prior to admission and of the way in which he plans to live when he is discharged. It is possible to plan nursing intelligently only if it is known how, from his point of view, it is desirable to live.

Most patients, if their illness permits, are willing to talk quite freely about the kind of house or flat they live in, the amenities or inconveniences of their place of residence, the neighbours, the shops, the other people in the household. Such conversation can remain completely neutral and yet allow the nurse to become aware of the patient's social standing, his attitude to neighbours of higher or lower social class, his views about the importance of pubs, cinemas and clubs in the neighbourhood, about schools, about the behaviour of children. The patient readily reveals his political outlook when he discusses the shortcomings of his local authority, for example in the matter of refuse collection or the provision of housing.

Without having asked any personal question at all a conversation which starts with such a topic as the patient's home can give a fairly good understanding of the patient's basic attitudes to a very wide range of experiences. A television programme for example can begin a conversation which explores the range and depth of the patient's education, of his interests in art, music, literature or theatre. Discussion of the newspapers not only has the value of keeping the patient informed and up to date but also touches on many opinions.

Politics and religion are topics which cannot really be avoided though some nurses endeavour to do so. These subjects are so important in most people's lives that any conversation attempting to circumvent them becomes artificial. There is no harm in hearing the patient's views or in stimulating him to further thought. These subjects only become difficult if the nurse's own views are so dogmatic, or if she is so emotional about them, that she cannot listen calmly to the patient. It is also important that the patient should feel completely free from pressure and that he should never come to think that his treatment might be jeopardized by the fact that his political or religious convictions are not those of a particular member of staff.

Most conversations, however apparently neutral the topic, tend to reveal some of the patient's specific difficulties. Although the nurse may not have asked a question she may soon become aware that the patient's political opinions have a delusional quality or that the topic of the educational system of the country is one about which husband and wife disagree, or that, although the patient's mother lives next door, she never visits. It is much better for information to be gradually pieced together than to press the patient for personal details.

While the nurse gets to know the patient, the patient learns a great deal about the nurse. Every occasion when nurse and patient are together offers as much opportunity to the patient as it does to the nurse. The nurse's tact, the genuineness of her interest, are among the personal characteristics the patient notices. Gestures, facial expression, tone of voice sometimes convey much more than actual words. A patient can usually judge if the nurse enjoys spending time with him or is merely doing so from a sense of duty. Any sign of impatience, of looking at the watch, is easily detected. Patients remember, often more readily than the nurse, what was talked about on the last occasion. If the nurse forgets, it is interpreted as a clear sign that she could not have been very interested, and this may be disappointing or even insulting to the patient. By contrast, to refer back to something the patient mentioned last time or to ask the patient about his activities on the day the nurse was off duty indicates interest.

A patient not only judges the nurse's behaviour to him

personally but also takes into account her behaviour to others. It is comforting to see another seriously disturbed patient competently and kindly dealt with and extremely worrying to see a nurse ignore someone in need of help or deal hastily with another patient. Each patient feels that the treatment meted out to another might easily happen to him and that any nurse who is inconsistent in her behaviour is not to be trusted.

Each patient's personal needs also determine the way in which he sees and uses the staff. A patient may find among the nurses one whose interest and concern he values and whom he hates at the same time for making him dependent on her. Another patient, feeling weak and insecure, develops a growing attachment to a nurse whose forceful personality he needs, while yet another treats the same nurse with hostility, rudeness and scorn, because he sees in her a representative of authority and he treats authority with his usual defiance and resentment. The patient's attitude to any one nurse may change during his stay in hospital, sometimes rapidly, sometimes over a period of time. It is usually interesting and worth while trying to find out what has caused changes in relationships, but this is not always possible to establish. Something in the nurse's tone of voice, her facial expression or her manner, may have conveyed to the patient disapproval or criticism, even if none was intended. Some reaction may not have been in keeping with the role which for the time being the nurse has fulfilled towards the patient. The patient may have expected protection and found that the nurse expected him to manage without it. He may have hoped for disapproval, but found the nurse non-committal. He may have expected affection and have felt rejected.

The ease with which nurse and patient establish contact depends to a large extent on personal characteristics of the people concerned. Patients and nurses of similar social class tend to find it easier to talk to each other than those whose social class background is very dissimilar.

The patient's age plays a part in interactions. Some nurses find older patients or very young patients easier to talk to than patients of their own age group.

It is often assumed that the presence of nurses of the opposite sex to the patients has beneficial effects on the atmosphere of the ward, but some patients may find it easier to converse with nurses of their own sex.

Nurse–patient interactions may change according to the function the nurse fulfils in the ward. The ward sister, as the head of the nursing team, more often represents a mother figure to the patients than does the junior nurse. She may be loved by some patients, hated by others, obeyed or defied according to each patient's previous experience. Her presence in the ward may help to reassure one patient, and cause anxiety to another. One patient may cling to her and seek her attention at all times, another avoid her whenever possible.

The nurse who has newly arrived in the ward may have to wait a few days before patients feel sufficiently comfortable with her to establish any contact. Some patients may, however, welcome the opportunity to offer guidance doing so, gain self-confidence and assert authority. Interaction between nurses and patients depends to some extent on the opportunities for frequent informal contact which arise. The architectural layout of the ward may facilitate such contact or render it difficult. Staffing problems and excessively large numbers of patients in the ward may make it more difficult to find occasions for informal chit-chat.

The more often nurses and patients see each other, the easier it becomes for patients to approach a nurse when the need for communications arise.

Not all interactions between nurses and patients exert an influence on the patient's recovery. Many contacts between nurse and patient merely serve to make the patient's stay more interesting, to reduce boredom or to convey to the patient a general sense of concern and interest in his welfare. A few interactions, however, lead to important developments in the patient's treatment. These arise from the nurse's sensitive appreciation of the patient's mood, preoccupation, and thought, gained during casual contact with the patient. Unless frequent interactions occur the opportunity for extended contact will be missed.

The patient's diagnosis affects the extent to which he chooses to make contact with nurses, and also the extent to which nurses choose to interact with the patient.

It would seem that depressed patients find it particularly difficult to approach nurses, though they experience the need for contact most. Nurses are often aware of the patient's isolation, yet have inhibitions in approaching the patient. It is sometimes difficult to feel that one has established contact with a patient suffering from schizophrenia, even though interactions may have taken place. Some patients suffering from neurotic disorders make their need for contact known; others however, are easily left out and ignored. Patients who have been in hospital for a long time may find their contact with nurses diminishing as the nurses whom they knew leave the ward to be replaced by others who devote their attention to newly admitted patients.

It seems important to offer some contact to all patients so that those whose need for interaction is greatest have the opportunity of having their need recognized. Contact with nurses for as prolonged a period as possible may become a vital factor in the progress of some of these patients. Deliberate and prolonged contact with patients makes great emotional demands on the nurse. She tries to help the patient without necessarily succeeding, or knowing whether her efforts are appreciated. Rejection by the patient is often very hurtful and it would be easy to withdraw, yet what the patient may need is acceptance and perseverance in spite of his rejecting attitude. To withdraw from contact may merely serve to reinforce the unhealthy pattern of interaction to which the patient is accustomed.

Even more difficult to tolerate than overt rejection is the silent apathy or the unemotional withdrawal of some patients. With such patients, the nurse has to learn the art of being with a patient without doing anything at all. Silence can be very uncomfortable. If one tries to make superficial conversation or fidgets or tries to encourage the patient to do things, he may become more and more tense. Quiet, relaxed, silent companionship may help the patient to realize that contact with people is safe.

It is not always easy to know whether touching is found to be helpful to the patient. When one feels sympathy or concern, when one wants to protect or comfort, one tends to touch people gently, hold hands, stroke the forehead. This may be appreciated, but some patients shrink from touch. It should then only be offered when the patient makes the first move. Some patients, on the other hand, seek closeness with the nurse. They try to cling, embrace, kiss or cuddle the nurse. It may then be the nurse who shrinks from such contacts and makes the patient feel rejected.

In conversation or in play the physical distance between nurse and patient may be important. Sometimes patients come very much closer to the person to whom they are speaking, than is usually the case among healthy people. Eye contact cannot be maintained when people get too close to each other; they then have to look past each other. It is possible that some patients find close bodily contact more tolerable than looking into the interlocutor's eyes.

The nurse's touch may convey a negative message. If, for example, the nurse touches the patient while he walks through a door it may almost seem like pushing. It would always seem advisable to observe how often, in the course of a day, a nurse touches a patient and to try and decide whether more or less touching is indicated. When more bodily contact seems desirable, physical care is often a good way of providing it. Bathing the patient, combing hair, rubbing the patient's back, massaging his hands, may be ways of offering bodily contact. Physical treatment, i.e. insulin treatment or continuous narcosis offers this opportunity.

During occupational or recreational periods occasions may arise when bodily contact can occur. Dancing for example or certain gymnastic exercises require that people hold each other's hands or help each other to turn or jump, give each other support to maintain equilibrium. In playing games, proximity to a nurse may be more acceptable to the patient if a table is between them than if they are sitting side by side.

The patient's difficulties in tolerating bodily contact, or in making excessive demands for it may have many reasons. One of these may be the arousal of sexual feelings. Another, especially in the case of patients suffering from schizophrenia, may be the patient's inability to create a satisfactory body image of himself. Educational influences and cultural background play an important part in determining the most comfortable way of making contact with people. The patient does not have to become consciously aware of the significance of what he is doing, but at times it may be helpful if he recognizes consciously any problem he may have in relation to physical closeness.

Most interactions between people involve talk. It is the nurse's function to enable the patient to talk as freely as possible. An interested, listening attitude, is a necessary beginning but it may not be enough. It may also be necessary to develop special techniques of communication. If the patient is to speak freely the place and the time must be right and the atmosphere conducive to talk. One cannot generalize about these factors. Sometimes sitting comfortably in armchairs is right but sitting down is not always necessary. Some patients can talk best while walking up and down the ward or the garden. Some patients talk when they are lying down in bed and the nurse sits beside them. Some patients can talk in the bath, others find that the best time to talk is over a meal or a cup of tea. Some patients can only talk freely if they are alone with the nurse, others don't mind talking in the presence of other people or may even need their presence to give them courage. Only very few patients feel able to talk seriously to a nurse as soon as the approach is made. A few patients feel under such pressure that they are constantly in search of a nurse who will listen. Most patients, however, need a period of superficial social chitchat before they can get to any important point they wish to make. Occasionally the patient can only speak about important matters at the very end of a period of interaction. When preparations for leave taking are obvious, the patient says: 'Oh just one more thing . . .' and then proceeds to talk about highly significant matters. Because this is known to happen, it is sometimes thought to be a good idea to tell the patient approximately how long the contact is likely to last. For example, it may be possible to say: 'I have half an hour now in which we can talk, then I shall have to attend to the medicine round' or 'I shall have to leave the ward at 5 p.m., we can go somewhere and talk until then.' It is also easier to sit with a patient in silence if both the nurse and the patient know in advance how much time is available. If a time limit is not set, there is a tendency to keep looking at one's watch and give the impression to the patient that one is longing to escape from contact with him.

Encouraging grunts and nods are often enough to keep the patient talking. Sometimes it is necessary to say a little more, 'Go on', 'Yes and then?', 'Tell me more', or 'I should like to hear more about this'. Acceptance of what the patient says as valuable, interesting and important helps the patient to continue. While the patient is talking he is sure to watch the nurse's face for signs of approval or disapproval. Neither approval nor disapproval help. As soon as the patient senses moral indignation, disapproval or condemnation, or as soon as he feels that he has hurt or embarrassed the nurse he is likely to stop talking.

If the nurse approves there is always the danger that sooner or later she will disapprove. For this reason the patient may be constantly on the alert to detect whether any disapproval might be forthcoming, and may in fact challenge or provoke the nurse to reject him, to disagree or to indicate her disapproval.

Sometimes nurses find quite spontaneously the right words and gestures, the right openings and responses, to make the patient feel at ease. More often though, what appears a commonsense reply to the nurse has the effect of convincing the patient that the nurse is no different from the lay people with whom he has talked before. Nurses who merely act on intuition and commonsense may find that their response has reinforced the reaction with which the patient had, previous to admission, met attempts to help him. The nurses' interaction with patients should develop into a purposive activity and the objectives for the patient should be clear.

Sometimes no more is required than to provide a sympathetic listener. One can indicate that one is such a listener by making observations about the patient's state of distress for example: 'I notice you are twisting your handkerchief . . . you appear tense . . . you seem to have been crying'. 'Would you like to talk about this?' 'Would it help you to tell me?' might be the kind of remarks which encourage a patient to talk more freely.

It sometimes helps to recognize how painful and distressing things must be for the patient. 'I can see that this makes you feel frightened' or 'This has made you feel lonely' may indicate the nurse's sympathy with the patient.

For some patients, the objective is to gain insight, for some to develop emotional control. It may help the patient if the nurse assists him to look at a problem more closely, to examine it from more points of view, and to express his thoughts more clearly.

If, for example, the patient talks about the attitude of his family it may help to ask the patient to describe it more fully or to say: 'And how does your sister feel about this?' or to explore a specific incident more fully by asking 'and then what did you say? . . . what did your sister say?'

To help the patient to gain emotional control it is sometimes useful to state how the situation is perceived by the nurse, e.g. 'You are angry' or 'You seem angry with me', or 'You are angry with me because I did not give in to you' or even 'I have the impression that you are doing this to make me angry'.

It is almost impossible to continue behaving in an uncontrolled manner once the difficulty has been recognized and openly stated.

Talking is not made easier by asking probing questions, either about the patient's life history or about his emotional difficulties or about his beliefs. Insight is not gained by asking 'Why'. If the patient knew why his behaviour is disturbed he would not need the nurse's help. He might discover 'why' if the nurse helps him to explore 'when, where, how, how long, what else, who with'.

Patients sometimes ask for advice. Advice is, however, rarely what the patient needs. Very often the patient who asks for advice merely wants someone to confirm that his own decision was the correct one.

It is hardly ever useful to give advice. If it were taken, the patient would place the responsibility for his action on the adviser, whereas the aim is to help the patient to make his own decison and himself to take responsibility for his own action. Advice given without due consideration of all relevant factors is useless, and conflicting advice undermines the patient's confidence in the staff and increases his difficulties. A nurse who gives advice too readily indicates to the patient that she considers herself competent to solve a problem which has proved to be a difficulty to him. This attitude may discourage him from further discussion of his conflicts, which he may feel are not taken seriously enough.

Of course, a straight refusal to give advice may be resented as is a refusal to answer direct questions. The nurse can avoid giving advice or answering questions by restating the problem, re-phrasing it, trying to get the patient to clarify it. A co-operative effort can be made to understand the full implication of any proposed action and to explore the patient's feelings about it. In the last resort the patient must feel free to make his own decisions, even his own mistakes.

Nurses are sometime tempted to use their knowledge of psychological mechanism to offer interpretation to the patient of varying depth and complexity. It is doubtful if such interpretation can be of help to the patient. Premature interpretation, even if correct, tends to be rejected and may render communication more difficult. When the patient is ready to accept interpretation, he has probably also gained sufficient insight to make his own interpretations. The patient may, for example, relate how his wife always pushes him around. The nurse may rightly interpret that the patient is trying to say: 'You are pushing me around in the same way as my wife does'. But it would not help to say to the patient: 'What you really mean is that I am pushing you around'. Insight is an experience which cannot be imposed.

During prolonged contact with a patient, interactions arise in which the nurse is uncertain how to respond.

Inevitably there are moments when her reply is tactless and she becomes aware of having offended the patient. Inevitably her response occasionally has the effect of cutting the patient off. Moments of guilt are bound to occur and there are periods of helplessness when nothing one says seems to make any difference and periods of frustration when the patient seems to be getting worse rather than better.

All nurses need the opportunity to discuss with others the interactions they have with patients. Some systematic inquiry is necessary at least at times which forces the nurse to recapitulate, if possible verbatim, what the patient said and did, what she said and did in response, and how the patient reacted.

Where several nurses interact with the same patient some comparison is necessary to learn from each other the different ways of dealing with similar problems and to gain an idea of the extent to which the patient's behaviour is the response to the way he is treated by different members of the staff. Discussion with other nurses is also needed to gain better understanding of the social factors involved in determining how people react to each other. A greater understanding of the complexity of human contact can be gained by a careful study of one's own contribution and experience.

Because prolonged contact with patients, particularly with those who need it most, causes stress to the nurse, supervision, frequent discussion and personal support is necessary for the nurse to retain her own emotional equilibrium, to gain increasing insight into her own problems, and to develop her therapeutic skills in relation to patients.

BOOKS FOR FURTHER READING

C. K. Aldrich. (1966) *An Introduction to Dynamic Psychiatry.* McGraw-Hill, New York.

G. Burton. (1965) *Nurse and Patient*. Tavistock, London.

S. H. Foulkes and E. Anthony. (1957) *Group Psychotherapy*. Penguin Books, Harmondsworth.

J. S. Hays and K. Larson. (1963) *Interacting with Patients*. Macmillan, New York.

H. E. Peplau. (1954) *Interpersonal Relations in Nursing*. Putnam, New York.

H. W. Render and M. O. Weiss. (1959) *Nurse-Patient Relationship in Psychiatry*. 2nd ed. McGraw-Hill, New York.

M. Weiss. (1954) *Attitudes in Psychiatric Nursing Care*. Putnam, New York.

CHAPTER 27

Relationships Within the Ward Community

In previous chapters it was shown that psychotherapy is a form of treatment in which the origins of the patient's problems are explored. It is largely concerned with the past.

Social therapy, by contrast, is concerned with the present. In daily contact with other people in the ward, the patient's problems are displayed. He may, for example, feel intense resentment regarding the way in which his mother has treated him. He talks, in his psychotherapeutic interview, of his mother's lack of understanding, of her aggressive attitude to him, of her preference for his brother. He may, in the ward, talk in a similar way about the ward sister. She too, he says, lacks understanding and sympathy, she too, dislikes him and shows preferences for other patients. It becomes clear to the doctor and the sister that he is 'projecting' on to the sister attitudes she does not really have, at least not at the outset of his stay in hospital.

In the ward it soon becomes obvious, however, that the patient's behaviour is so hostile and provocative towards the ward sister that before long her attitude may well be as he describes. He does not at first realize the part that he himself plays in creating unfavourable attitudes in other people. In the ward the other patients and the staff can confront him with the effect his own behaviour has on others. When he begins to see how he himself creates antagonism in others he may begin to reflect that he might have provoked his mother in a similar way. He may gain a deeper understanding of his past problems from an investigation of his current ones, just as an awareness of his past attitudes may help him to understand his present ones.

In social therapy use is made of the fact that everyone —staff and patients—acts as observer and as participant in the interactions that take place. Jointly, they are often in a much better position to understand what the interactions mean, than are the individual participants of such interactions.

Patients may be able to observe that even the apparently private relationship between one nurse and one patient affects the ward community as a whole. Many of the patients' difficulties affect not only attitudes to staff but also attitudes to each other. Hostilities, friendships, close attachments between patients are important to everybody. The way in which some patients make a bid for prominence and leadership, the way in which rivalries and jealousies develop and are dealt with, the way in which one patient is helped by another, or the way in which someone is rebuffed or hurt, are all crucial to the feelings of every single member of the ward community. Social therapy is an attempt to manipulate the environment in order to produce change in the patient's behaviour and to use to the fullest possible extent the contributions of all staff and all patients in a treatment plan.

Patients can only learn to contribute effectively if the general climate of the ward permits them to use their initiative and their judgement, and if they have freedom to express their opinion. They need the opportunity to make decisions and to deal with the problems which arise as a result of their decisions.

Whether a hospital can provide the patient with such an environment depends to a large extent on the nursing staff. Nurses are sometimes found to be so authoritarian in outlook and action that patients are given very little opportunity to exercise their initiative. Nurses tend to decide what is good for the patient and tell them how to behave. Nurses who behave in an authoritarian way often do so because they themselves are members of a hospital organization which is authoritarian in outlook. Nurses in the ward tend to be low in the hierarchical arrangement of the hospitals. Orders from above may reach them without explanation or opportunity for discussion. They gain approval from those in senior positions if they carry out orders smoothly. They, in turn, give instructions to patients and expect them to be carried out smoothly.

If patients are to take responsibility nurses also need to feel free to make decisions and to accept authority.

Free and open communication is only possible for patients if nurses can communicate freely with other members of the staff. Mutual understanding and respect are essential ingredients of successful staff co-operation. These grow gradually and slowly. There are many obstacles to understanding which must be patiently removed. The tradition of some psychiatric hospitals is against free speech from nurses in the presence of doctors. Where formerly the Medical Superintendent reigned supreme it is hard for doctors to exchange opinions freely, let alone for nurses to offer theirs. Traditionally nursing is arranged in an hierarchical order which may be a hindrance to free expression of opinions.

Staff Meetings

A programme of re-education of all staff members may be necessary to enable them to use social therapy effectively. Frequent staff meetings have become an essential part of the organization of most psychiatric hospitals. The mere arrangement of staff meetings, however, is not sufficient to ensure that they are of use to all concerned. Sometimes nurses find it difficult to speak at meetings and they keep information to themselves which might have been of great value had it been shared. Junior nurses, particularly, find it very hard to talk in the presence of their seniors, especially if they feel in some way critical of a senior. Again, nurses may find it hard to speak freely before doctors or social workers. Antagonism between any two members of the staff may make it very difficult for them to discuss any topic objectively and unemotionally. In any discussion about patients, personal feelings tend to become obvious to others and it is understandable that the individual should try to protect himself from exposure. Silence may be one way of achieving protection. Apparently free discussion, but of trivial points, is another device.

In any discussion the opinion of an individual may not be well received by the others; there is, moreover, always the danger that such an opinion may be wrong or that it may seem silly to others. There is no way of finding out except by risking exposure, but exposure may be uncomfortable and therefore there is a tendency to try to avoid it. Staff meetings inevitably have their painful moments. It is part of the professional growth of each nurse to learn to deal with her own emotions, whether they are aroused by colleagues or by patients. Every difficult experience during a staff meeting can help her to gain more understanding of the interaction which takes place among people and of the way in which attitudes can be modified.

Ward Meetings

The chief instrument of social therapy is the meeting of patients for the purpose of solving the problems of communal living. Patients must have the chance to solve genuine problems which resemble those of real life which patients are likely to lead after discharge.

The patients' physical environment needs to be under the patients' control. If the ward resembles a luxury hotel or an airport lounge, life in the ward takes on an unreal quality and feelings of transience and detachment prevail. Patients feel that no decisions need to be taken because the ward cannot possibly have any personal meaning for them. When there is overcrowding in the ward and squalor in the environment no decisions can be taken by the patients which can make any difference to their quality of living.

Some identification with the hospital and with the ward in particular is necessary. It is useful to observe how the possessive pronoun is used in the wards. If the ward sister refers to *my* ward she is likely to be the person who makes decisions about choice of furniture, arrangement of ornaments, spending of money on equipment. In some hospitals the matron or the assistant matron makes these decisions and refer to the wards as 'my wards' and to the nurses as 'my staff'. Where social therapy is being used the patients need to feel that the ward is 'theirs'. *They* decide about the character of their personal environment, arrange personal property and make responsible decisions about the maintenance, repair and replacement of furnishings and equipment. Patients show visitors around their ward. They explain the ward to new patients. They take pride in the appearance of the ward, or feel embarrassment if visitors call when the ward is untidy.

Meetings of patients can be used to define the extent to which patients feel responsible for their environment. If they do not feel responsible, they will interpret any shortcomings as evidence of insufficient concern for their well-being. 'They' are blamed for not providing all that is needed. 'They' won't give us ashtrays, 'they' are slow in carrying out repairs, 'they' don't seem to care! 'They'—the authorities'—are never clearly identified. As long as they can be blamed, patients can remain passive, and avoid looking at their own problems. As soon as patients begin to ask 'How can *we* solve this problem?' or 'What can *I* do to help to solve it?' or '*Whose* problem is this, is it my own?', some useful exercises in decision-making follow.

Patients in their meetings can deal with decisions about the way their life is arranged. They may decide that something needs to be done to make arrangements better known or more comprehensible. Calendars may be necessary to ensure that everyone is clearly orientated. Clocks may be needed to help people synchronize their activities. Signposting may facilitate movement around the hospital.

Some structure can be imposed by agreeing on time-tables. Arrangements of events can be made known on notice-boards, in bulletins or through the medium of a news-sheet. Patients can control the amount of contact they have with each other by allocating certain rooms for television viewing, others for silent occupations, others for social gatherings. Arrangements of chairs around the fireplace or around small coffee tables will help to establish contact in small groups.

Patients can be responsible for making and enforcing rules necessary for communal living. Patients learn very easily to cope with their own deviant members, and they benefit from the experience of having authority.

The distribution of the work of the hospital is the business of patients' meetings. Every task that can be organized or performed by patients should be. Nurses and patients work together, but patients decide what is the nurses' share of the work and what their own. Arrangements for bedmaking, sweeping, dusting, washing up, can be left entirely to patients in some wards. Decisions about times for getting up or for going to bed, for the hours of use of radiogram, wireless and television, can be reached without staff intervention. Preparation for evening entertainments, provision of refreshments, invitations to patients in other wards are examples of the kinds of activities which patients can take over. The purpose of patients' activities should always be clear. It should never be a matter of 'helping the staff' but rather of 'patients' responsibilities' with which staff help only when a patient's illness makes this necessary. Responsibility is usually accompanied by difficulties and frustrations and these should be shouldered by the patients themselves.

If the cleanliness of the ward is the patients' responsibility, they must find ways of dealing with those who do not pull their weight, they must suffer the discomfort of living in a ward which has not been cleaned, they must bear the criticism of outside authority, for example, the Hospital Committee, if the ward is dirty. Each of these frustrations can become the topic for discussion at a ward meeting, sometimes in a general kind of way, for example by examining what is meant by sense of responsibility and how it is acquired, or in a specific way, for example by discussing a particular patient who will not do his share of the work in spite of all the different approaches tried by the other members of the group.

No decision is permanent. The ward community is complex and constantly changing. The patients are constantly provided with new problems to solve.

There are many possible methods of involving patients in discussions. In some instances the entire ward population meets once a week. In other hospitals meetings are held daily and include as many of the patients and staff as are able to be present at the time. In some instances group meetings take place several times each day but the composition of the group and the purpose of the meetings differ.

When meetings are held infrequently, for example once per week, they tend to deal with administrative routine aspects of ward life. Ward chores may be arranged and entertainments or outings organized. Patients may be able to discuss difficulties encountered in community living, for example the fact that the television set is used too noisily or that some patients feel the need for a quiet place for reading. The value of occupational therapy may come under scrutiny. Quite often the quality of the food is raised for discussion and at times hospital rules are questioned. It is possible to conduct meetings of this kind quite informally, without an agenda and without an official chairman, or alternatively patients may wish to arrange a more formal opening of the meeting, by keeping records of business, reading or circulating minutes and preparing an agenda.

There may be value in both kinds of meeting. If the opening phase is left entirely unstructured there may be some initial silence which may then lead to tension and consequently to some very significant topic being raised. At the same time this may frighten some patients who may find it difficult to make the effort to attend. Some patients may hesitate in these circumstances to speak or bring up their points of view because they feel sure that all other business is more important and because they themselves feel so insecure and insignificant.

A more formally conducted meeting may have the advantage of making a definite place on the agenda for business raised at other times by the more diffident patients. It also gives the opportunity for practising the holding of office and patients can elect their chairman and secretary. A great deal of what needs to be said will, however, never be raised at all at a formally conducted meeting because there never seems to be a right time and place for it.

When meetings are held infrequently content rarely goes beyond factual business. By the time feelings between patients are overtly aroused there is often insufficient time left to discuss these fully and to help each person to understand and cope with them. The meeting closes at a point of high tension and what happens after the meeting becomes the really important factor. The next meeting is too far away to allow feelings to remain unresolved, so immediately after the meeting nurses may try to help the patient who is disturbed, or patients, over their cup of tea or in various corners in the ward, themselves deal with the feelings of which they have become aware. The meeting may have served the purpose of making everyone more aware of a problem; the solution of the problem takes place elsewhere. The following meeting begins without reference to the previous one though the continuity may become obvious by the way everyone studiously avoids raising another emotionally charged topic.

If meetings are infrequent it is difficult to discuss difficulties between patients and staff. Although often patients may wish to criticize staff, they may not venture to do so overtly. Consequently criticism of staff may often only be implied. For example, talk about hospital rules may really imply criticism of those who made them; talk of disturbance caused by a patient may include hints that the nurses ought to have prevented it. If patients are to explore freely their feelings about staff, meetings need to be held fairly frequently.

Not only the frequency of meetings, but also their size and composition determine how meetings are used. If very large numbers of patients are present it is impossible for everyone to speak. The silent members are less conspicuous than they would be in a smaller group. New members can join the group unobtrusively and can gradually gain confidence as they listen to a number of people speak

On the other hand, in a very large meeting it is impossible for everyone to sit face to face. It is easy to remain outside the group and to be overlooked altogether. Patients in a large meeting always outnumber staff. In some ways this can make it clearly a patients' meeting, but it can also lead to a very conspicuous dominance by any member of staff who assumes leadership.

If the number of patients is small any person who absents himself from the meeting is at once seen not to be present, whether he remains away altogether or whether he is physically there but chooses to remain silent. In a small meeting it is possible to become aware of every person in the group. Not only what people say, but also their facial expression, their way of sitting in the chair, their sidelong glances at other people, their fidgeting, smoking or mannerisms become important. There is no way of disguising their attitudes to each other and consequently every person's awareness of tensions in the ward is heightened and every person feels conspicuous in the group. When there are few patients the staff ratio is often relatively high and it becomes necessary for the staff to join in if they do not wish to create the appearance of a split between patients and staff.

In small groups feelings are frequently discussed because they cannot be covered up so easily even if speech is avoided. How freely patients can express their own feelings, how safely they can involve the staff and how constructively they can use group meetings, depends largely on the level of understanding reached by the staff.

Meetings can be used to make decisions about the way in which patients spend their time. Because the patients themselves make the decisions and because decisions are reached publicly they have a reasonable chance of being carried out. On the other hand failure to carry out a decision can become a topic of discussion. Many patients have special difficulties in carrying out their own decisions. They benefit from seeing the effect their behaviour has on others and also from realizing that other people have similar difficulties.

Life in hospital should offer all possible opportunities for the patients' difficulties to become overt. Living in a relatively confined space with a number of other people, all of whom are difficult, is inevitably frustrating and tension-producing. Patients who are inconsiderate to others, for example, inevitably demonstrate this early on and soon other patients comment on the effect this has on them. Any attempt to change, to show more consideration for others, is also noticed and the patient learns by direct experience the pleasure of receiving other people's approval. In meetings patients learn to recognize other people's strongly held values. Other people's comments mirror back varied aspects of the patients' own personality.

In hospital the patient needs the opportunity to shoulder responsibility for a job and if being unreliable is one of his problems he needs a chance to demonstrate how and why it is difficult for him to perform his allotted task. The annoyance of the other patients at being let down is part of the necessary treatment. Knowing that the difficulties are understood and being given repeated opportunities to try again help to make progress.

There are some events in the ward for which patients can assume partial responsibility but where the staff cannot ultimately divest themselves of their share. It is for example useful that all patients should be concerned if one member of the group attacks another. Everyone may feel in some way responsible because they did nothing to prevent the outburst. Someone may have been particularly aware of the rising anxiety but failed to draw the nurse's attention to it. Someone may feel that he has contributed to the incident by his own un-friendly attitude to the patient. It is the business of all others to try to understand the aggressive feeling of the patient, while at the same time becoming more aware of similar feelings in themselves. Fear, anger, irritation, guilt, sympathy, are common ground for patients and staff in the ward. The ultimate responsibility for pro-tecting the patients from the effect of violence remains that of the staff, and patients need to know how far they can rely on staff to carry out their duty. Ward meetings are good opportunities to clarify the feelings between patients and staff with regard to such points.

The term 'therapeutic community' has been used to describe a hospital where every aspect of community life is planned to serve a therapeutic aim. Group discussions are an essential part of a therapeutic community but they serve their purpose only if there is worth-while community life and if the staff have developed attitudes in which they can accept each patient as a full member of a therapeutic team.

Although the patients in a therapeutic community adopt functions and responsibilities which, in different settings, belong to members of the staff, there are certain specific roles which belong to the staff.

The staff are the more permanent members of the community. Patients leave the hospital as they improve. The staff are responsible for the growth of a specific culture within the hospital. The culture of a therapeutic community is one in which equality is highly valued. Relationships change in such a way that people feel increasingly confident of each other. Every effort is made to blur not only the role distinction between different categories of staff but also between staff and patients. The universal use of Christian names may contribute to the realization of role fusion.

This fusion of roles, however desirable, produces certain stress at times. Staff members may find it difficult to discount entirely the specific skills acquired before they started to work in a therapeutic community.

Doctors, social workers, occupational therapists and nurses may rightly feel that their training enables them to make specific contributions to the community. Their different level of remuneration, their membership of different professional organizations may render it difficult for them to operate realistically in an egalitarian setting.

A therapeutic community which has been in existence for a period of time develops norms of behaviour which may not be relevant to the culture outside the hospital. For this reason, however therapeutic the cultural values of the community may be, criticisms from outside are common. Those who belong to a therapeutic community are often accused of being too 'permissive'. New staff members may for a time share the standards of the outside community, and fail to understand the objectives of the therapeutic community. The established staff may find the new staff members too 'judgemental', too 'authoritarian' or too 'custodial'.

The duty of the staff is to interpret the therapeutic community in an unambiguous way to the outside and to mediate between the demands and interpretations of the outside community and the patients.

People who work and live with each other develop an understanding which makes communication easy, even if a great deal is left unsaid. People's tone of voice is understood, their background is known, shared experience is referred to without it being made explicit and understanding of each other's difficulties is taken for granted. Psychological insight is achieved in co-operative exploration and as a result of cumulative experience.

Conversation between people who know each other well often becomes unintelligible to outsiders. New patients and new members of staff may find the experience of entering such a community profoundly unsettling because they cannot understand the hints, the jargon and the ambiguous statements which established members use in communication. Making the environment explicit to new patients in a friendly unambiguous way is the function of the staff.

Social therapy is a form of treatment which is of value to patients suffering from a wide variety of disorders. Some psychiatrists see this form of treatment of special value in schizophrenia, to counteract the patient's tendency to become isolated. The patient's problems of identity confusion and disorder of ego boundary can be most effectively attacked by social therapy. Some neurotic patients find the experience of value. Co-operation with others, exercise of authority, and practice in assuming responsibility enhances the patient's self-respect. Participation in group activities and discussion with patients and staff helps to develop insight and promotes emotional growth.

Social therapy is of particular value to patients suffering from personality disorders. Patients suffering from psychopathic disorder do not respond easily to any other form of treatment. Their distrust of authority and their general antisocial attitudes make it difficult for them to accept treatment of any other kind and to persevere with it. In a therapeutic community these patients are submitted to the control of other patients like themselves; they may learn to conform to the rules imposed by members of their own group, when they might reject any standards which staff members might try to promote.

Patients suffering from alcoholism and from drug addiction may also be more able to function in a group of people who, they think, can understand them. They feel that, generally, doctors and nurses and the community as a whole are unsympathetic.

Special units for the treatment of specific personality disorders acquire a separate deviant culture pattern shared eventually by patients and staff. The kind of life which is led in such a community may acquire for the patients a worthwhileness which they may be unwilling to give up. Return to the wider community may be all the more difficult if patients have accepted the hospital culture as desirable and satisfying.

There are certain elements in the use of social therapy which are universally applicable. The environment in which the patient lives can be used to give him the support he needs for security and the freedom he needs for development. The way in which the patient spends his time can provide problems which must be solved.

The patient has experience of belonging to a group; he learns to co-operate with people and finds people who can help him to develop new modes of behaviour. He meets staff members whose behaviour is different from the authoritarian approach he has met before. The staff participate fully in the corporate life of the community, but they represent the normal non-deviant world. They help to form a bridge for the patient to cross when he is ready to leave hospital.

Books for Further Reading

D. H. Clark. (1964) *Administrative Therapy*. Tavistock, London.

J. Cumming and E. Cumming. (1964) *Ego and Milieu*. Tavistock, London.

M. Jones. (1952) *Social Psychiatry*. Tavistock, London.

D. V. Martin. (1962) *Adventures in Psychiatry*. Bruno Cassirer, Oxford.

R. N. Rapoport. (1961) *Community as Doctor*. Tavistock, London.

CHAPTER 28

Notes on Classification and on Some Mental Disorders

CLASSIFICATION of illness is useful in so far as it helps to clarify ideas about the nature of the disorder and to aid its treatment. The first step in classification is usually to give a detailed *description* of the form various disorders take at a given moment and during the whole of their course. Certain groups of symptoms, or syndromes, are often given particular names. The *descriptive* form of classification may lead to knowledge about the *location* of the disorder, e.g. the heart and the liver, the brain or 'the mind', if no other location can be found, and may help to provide understanding of the *causation* of the illness. The more that is known about the cause of illness, the more useful the classification, because, by these means, more specific treatment can be developed.

Descriptive classification is the one most used in the case of mental disorders. Many psychiatric symptoms, such as restlessness, overactivity, refusal of food, and insomnia must be treated. Nursing care can be planned more easily if it is possible to predict what symptoms are liable to arise, so that a knowledge of the more common psychiatric syndromes is helpful.

There is no *location* to be found in most mental illness, but in some forms of these disorders a physical cause is known to exist; for instance, the organic lesion may be situated in the brain. In other disorders, mental symptoms may be associated with generalized infection of toxaemia, and treatment of the organic disorder leads to improvement in the mental condition. But the mental disorder is neither specifically the result of an organic illness nor located in an organ. Some forms of mental disorder, those termed functional, do not appear to have any organic basis whatever. Research is being carried out in this field because many psychiatrists feel convinced that ultimately an organic disturbance will be found in all forms of mental illness. So far, however, there is little to show in the way of conclusive results.

Investigation into the *causes* of mental illness is not as rewarding and is much more complex than it is in the case of physical disorders. Usually some immediate precipitating cause is found which the patient considers to be 'the' cause of the illness. Physical illness may be considered as being a precipitating cause of mental disorder. Occasionally a patient, prior to his mental illness, has suffered a disaster of such magnitude that it appears wholly reasonable to attribute the breakdown to stress. Frequently, however, mental illness is attributed to events which appear so trivial that there is a compulsion to seek further explanation as to why the patient should have reacted so abnormally to the situation. Heredity and early childhood experiences may partially explain why he should have been predisposed to mental disorder. Knowledge of his personality make-up before the illness may also help understanding of the particular form which the disorder has taken. On the whole it is more useful to think not of illness that has befallen a hitherto healthy person, but rather of people who, as a result of a combination of circumstances, are reacting abnormally to stress situations.

Various patterns of abnormal reaction can be described. The form which may be taken by any individual patient's mental disorder appears to depend on constitutional factors, including heredity, physique and endocrine balance. Early upbringing may determine his vulnerability to stress.

Treatment consists in assessing the relative importance of the various causes of the patient's breakdown and acting accordingly. If excessive stress is responsible for the breakdown of a hitherto well-adjusted person, treatment may consist in providing rest and support while the patient recovers and in endeavouring to prevent further excessive stress. A patient who is constitutionally weak must be helped to learn how to live with his disability and how to avoid excessively stressful situations. If upbringing and education appear to be at fault the patient may be helped to retrace his steps and to develop into a better-adapted person. A detailed knowledge and understanding of the patient's background and personality may be more helpful in psychiatry than any attempt at naming a specific disease.

There are many different classifications in use at the present time. None of these is entirely satisfactory and no attempt is made here to classify; only a brief description is given of some of the disorders with which nurses are most commonly concerned. A textbook of psychiatry should be consulted for details of various psychiatric conditions.

MENTAL DISORDERS ASSOCIATED WITH ORGANIC DISEASES

(a) *Psychosomatic disorders* are conditions in which physical symptoms are noticeably related to emotional disturbances.

The following examples are not uncommon.

Asthmatic attacks are frequently precipitated by periods of emotional stress and may cease when the patient feels relaxed and happy.

Vascular disorders, particularly congestion of the mucous membranes of the respiratory tract, are aggravated by anxiety. Fainting is associated with excitement and fear.

Hypertension and coronary occlusion occur more frequently in people who are of a tense and worrying disposition. Hyperthyroidism, ulcerative colitis, peptic ulcers, urticaria and migraine, are all conditions which tend to respond better to treatment when the patient's emotional adjustment is taken into account. The symptoms are not entirely due to psychological difficulties but improvement often coincides with improvement in the patient's mental state.

(b) *Infective exhaustive psychoses or toxic confusional states* occur during infections and sometimes last much longer than the infective illness. The infection may involve the central nervous system, but toxins produced by micro-organisms in other parts of the body are often held to be responsible. Confusional symptoms can occur in such varied conditions as metabolic disorders, endocrine disorders, drug intoxication, alcoholism, anoxaemia of heart failure, hypoglycaemia, uraemia and metal poisoning. Confusional syndromes very commonly occur in puerperal psychoses.

The most prominent symptoms are clouding of consciousness, disorientation for time and place and disturbance of memory for recent events. The patient is unable to understand what is happening around him. His attention wanders; consequently his memory appears faulty. He misidentifies people and often fails to recognize familiar objects. His actions may appear strange because he may carry out correct movements but in the wrong circumstances; e.g. he may try to write with a cigarette, or eat soap, because he is unable to identify the objects he is using. Movements appear purposive. Often the patient's usual occupational activities are repeated. He may have hallucinatory experiences. He may see terrifying visions, or behave as if he were responding to voices. In some conditions he feels small animals crawling over the skin or describes minute moving visual hallucinatory experiences. Following some infections the cardinal symptoms are tiredness, irritability and depression. Whenever the picture is one of infective exhaustive psychosis it is important by means of careful examination, to establish a diagnosis of the physical disorder.

Treatment is aimed at conserving the patient's strength and improving his physical condition by attention to diet, fluid balance and oral hygiene, and the prevention of secondary infection and exhaustion. Bed rest is often essential. The patient's restlessness and inability to co-operate because he fails to understand or remember instructions must be taken into account.

(c) *Dementia* occurs when there is permanent damage of the brain tissue. Cerebral arteriosclerosis, cerebral syphilis, brain tumours, head injuries, prolonged effect of drugs, poisons (particularly carbon monoxide and alcohol) and irreversible hypoglycaemia may all cause permanent organic and mental changes. Dementia also accompanies degenerative changes which occur in some apparently hereditary conditions, e.g. Huntington's chorea and any type of pre-senile dementia.

Dementia may be described as a failing of intellectual ability. The patient's performance in intelligence tests deteriorates, although his vocabulary remains good. He becomes unable to use symbols in thinking. Abstract thought becomes difficult, but the patient retains the ability to solve concrete problems, e.g. he may be unable to perform an addition using figures, but able to do it if he has beads. He may be unable to say how he would share a sum of money among several people, but actually do it correctly if given the money. He may be unable to experience emotional bonds with people not actually present. He may show tenderness to his wife when she is beside him, but appear to be unconcerned about her in her absence.

The patient becomes increasingly unable to vary his responses. He can see only one way of doing things and cannot modify his reactions. In psychological tests this is shown by the way in which he classifies objects; e.g. if he is given differently shaped objects of different colours he may classify either according to colour or to shape. Once he has done this he finds it impossible to change the classification. Such disability in daily life might tend to make the patient irritable and apparently stubborn. His mood varies rapidly—tears and laughter are easily aroused. His understanding of other people's actions and particularly of other people's feelings declines. Therefore he may appear self-centred and uninhibited. His relations may notice a decline in moral standards. Progressive dementia ultimately leads to complete helplessness and dependence.

Nursing care is concerned primarily with the preservation of physical health. Although the patient may eventually become bedridden this should be delayed as long as possible. Good nursing care can be effective also in delaying deterioration in habits and in helping the patient to remain socially adapted and as active as possible. A great deal of suffering can be spared to the patient and his relatives if his appearance is well preserved and he remains socially acceptable for the longest possible time.

PERSONALITY DISORDERS

The term 'psychopathic personality' is used to describe a form of personality disorder affecting the patient's emotional and social adjustment to other people. Patients who are called 'psychopaths' are not suffering from mental illness, yet their conduct is so abnormal that they must be considered as being mentally disordered.

Not all asocial or antisocial people can be considered

to be psychopathic. In the Mental Health Act some attempt was made to define the concept, but it remains difficult to establish generally acceptable criteria. Many psychiatrists therefore prefer to refrain from using the diagnosis of 'psychopathic disorder'.

The disturbance dates from a very early age, and one of its characteristics is a failure to learn from experience. The psychopathic patient is immature in every aspect of his behaviour. He is impulsive, lacks foresight, is unable to persevere in his endeavours or to postpone gratification of his desires. He may have had frequent changes of jobs, given up some because of differences of opinion with other people, lost others because of his inability to conform to discipline.

Some psychopathic people are highly gifted, but their instability prevents achievement of real success. Although many psychopathic people are friendly, often charming, they lack emotional depth and are unable to form lasting friendships.

Psychopathic people are often unhappy people, who may seek solace in drink or drugs, or may drift into sexual perversion, prostitution or crime.

In the course of the patient's unhappy life he may seek psychiatric help and may agree to admission to a psychiatric hospital. After a short period, however, he may find restrictions irksome, people uncongenial, and may take his discharge before effective treatment is possible.

During his stay in hospital the patient can be helped if he can feel that he is accepted by some member of the staff, and if he can establish satisfying emotional relationships with somebody. This can best be achieved in a ward or hospital where a 'therapeutic community' can be created. The patients assume responsibility with the staff for the functioning of the ward, and for the treatment of each member of the community. They develop interest and understanding of each others' problems, become more interested, more tolerant of difficult behaviour. As they come to feel accepted by the others their behaviour improves and they learn to form closer personal bonds.

With advancing years most psychopathic patients settle down to a more satisfactory pattern of living.

NEUROTIC DISORDERS

Generally speaking the neuroses are those disorders in which the patient's failure in adaptation is partial rather than complete. It is unusual for neurotic disorders to become so severe that continuation of life in the community becomes impossible, or that the patient becomes a danger to himself or others. Hallucinations and delusions do not usually occur in neurotic disorders and, although these conditions are responsible for a tremendous amount of suffering, there are relatively few neurotic patients in psychiatric hospitals. This is due partly to the fact that some hospitals are so overcrowded that they have difficulty in making beds available for these patients and partly to the fact that many neurotic patients derive more benefit from out-patient treatment than from in-patient care.

Only the most severely disturbed neurotic patients, those who are unable to be cared for in the community, are likely to be accepted into a psychiatric hospital. There are, however, increasing numbers of special units for in-patient treatment of neurotic disorders where psychotherapeutic and environmental influences are brought to bear on the patient and where physical treatment is available when it is required.

In neurotic disorders constitutional factors appear to be partly responsible in rendering the patient particularly vulnerable to stress. It is usually possible, however, to demonstrate also that the illness is in some way related to traumatic experiences and to the parental attitude towards the patient in early childhood.

The neurotic symptoms are related to conflict. They are an indication of the patient's inability to solve a conflict on a conscious basis. On an unconscious level, they may serve to solve the conflict situation, although not in a very successful way.

(a) Anxiety States

This is a most distressing condition in which the patient experiences intense feeling of 'anxiety' and presents in exaggerated form all the physical symptoms which normally accompany any feeling of fear or apprehension in preparation for action.

The patient complains of feeling worried and afraid, but does not know of what. He anticipates the worst, feels that some action is required, but does not know what such action should be. At times his feelings amount to 'panic attacks'. He is restless, his muscle tone is increased, sometimes tremors are present. His pulse is rapid and his blood pressure raised. His mouth is dry, the palms of his hands often perspire, and beads of perspiration may appear on his forehead. He complains of headache, nausea and often also of frequency of micturition.

The patient's anxiety is not related to any adequate conscious cause, but often he becomes aware of the physiological changes which have taken place, and believes himself to be physically ill. He interprets his palpitations as evidence of heart disorder, or his nausea as evidence of carcinoma of the stomach. He may then explain to himself and others that his anxiety is caused by his physical illness.

Anxiety results in increased output of energy. As the patient's fear of physical disease increases, his nausea, and possibly also diarrhoea, lead to a diminished intake of food and consequently his physical condition often suffers. He may lose weight and become seriously undernourished. Sleep is usually disturbed and he may have difficulty in going off to sleep and may wake repeatedly during the night. The patient may be intensely irritable and easily disturbed by noise. He may be acutely aware of his abnormal state of mind and be afraid of losing grip and of becoming insane.

The treatment depends on the existing circumstances and how far these can be modified, and on the extent to which the cause is rooted in the past. It is necessary to consider how far the patient's earlier childhood experiences have contributed to the development of his attitude, and how far back it is necessary to retrace steps in order to help him proceed along healthier lines.

The patient's physical condition must be considered first of all. Only after a very thorough physical examination can he be effectively persuaded that he is physically healthy. To some patients this is reassuring, others find it difficult to accept the fact that the symptoms could have psychogenic causes. Some explanation of the physiology of stress may then be helpful.

Sedation in some form, may be helpful in producing relaxation, while psychotherapy may help the patient to a better understanding of his problems. Continuous narcosis or modified insulin therapy may be necessary when his physical condition is poor.

Nurses can contribute to the patient's recovery by remaining calm, and emotionally unaffected by the patient's anxiety. They may be able to communicate to him a feeling of security, which is often lacking in his home background. Sympathetic listening may have the effect of helping such a patient to see his own problems in better perspective by the verbalizing of his fears and anxieties. The mere presence of a calm person whom he knows well may have a soothing effect on him.

(b) Obsessive-Compulsive Disorders

This is one of the most incapacitating mental disorders. Patients who, prior to their illness, have often been known for their reliability, trustworthiness and meticulous neatness, during their illness show these traits in exaggerated form, so much so that they become aware of the absurd nature of their compulsive actions but are unable to desist without becoming severely anxious.

Sometimes a patient becomes preoccupied with some thought or phrase, occasionally of an obscene or blasphemous nature, considered totally alien to his character. Nevertheless the thought persistently intrudes into consciousness and no amount of will-power can rid him of it.

Some patients find, with increasing frequency, that they are in doubt whether an action just completed was correctly performed and feel obliged to repeat it. After checking, the patient still feels doubtful and so repeats the action again. He may be fully aware of the fact that his doubts are without foundation. Often such a compulsive action develops into a ritual which is carried out in precisely the same manner on each occasion and is then repeated, lest a mistake has occurred. The patient becomes intensely worried, feeling that something terrible may happen if the ritual is not correctly performed.

Some patients are terrified of going out, of crossing the street, of heights or bridges, or of being in an enclosed space. Some patients are afraid of knives or sharp instruments, always recognizing that these fears are irrational.

The patient's symptoms may give an indication of the underlying conflict. Fear of heights may be associated with an unconscious desire on the part of the patient to throw himself over; fear of knives may be found in one who is afraid of hurting people and who may be protecting himself from his own unconscious impulses to do so. Hand-washing and the expressed wish to be scrupulously clean may represent the patient's attempt to rid himself of a feeling of being unclean. A feeling of guilt about some real or imagined wrong-doing, often of a sexual nature, may, without the patient's awareness of the connection, be expressed by an exaggerated concern about dirt.

Patients who develop obsessional neuroses are some-times found to have been subjected to very rigorous and early habit training. The parents may have been rigid, methodical and overconscientious people who may have made excessive demands for early socialization and their own rigid moral standards may have been taken over by the patient. To what extent the parents' person-ality is transmitted genetically, predisposing the patient to an obsessional illness, or to what extent the mode of training is responsible for producing the obsessional personality pattern is not always clear.

Only the most severely handicapped of these patients are likely to be admitted to hospital as in-patients. Many obsessional patients, in spite of the suffering they may undergo, succeed in remaining gainfully employed. The severity of the symptoms fluctuates with environ-mental circumstances.

During periods of stress the patient's rituals may become complicated and so extensive that he is quite incapable of keeping them under control. It may take him all his time to wash and dress, so that he never reaches his place of work, or at work he may feel com-pelled to go over each item so often that very little is done and he is unable to hold down his job. Sometimes, although the compulsive symptoms remain relatively mild, the anxiety associated with attempting to control them is so great that the patient's symptoms on admis-sion to hospital are those of a severe anxiety state.

Treatment and nursing depend largely on the severity of the symptoms. In the calm and relatively well-ordered atmosphere of the hospital ward these are likely to become less intolerable. The fewer the demands made on the patient the more likely he will be to become more relaxed. On the other hand, discussion of emotional conflicts may lead to a temporary exacerbation, but the patient may benefit ultimately from a better understanding of his problems.

It has been found that patients suffering from obsessional neurosis do not respond to psychotherapy. More consideration is therefore given to the rehabilitation of the patient, and treatment is aimed at reducing environmental stress and helping him to learn to live more successfully, in spite of his compulsive symptoms.

If the compulsive acts in themselves are relatively mild and not harmful, the patient may be helped to reduce his anxiety about them and to live a comparatively normal life. If the compulsive acts are seriously incapacitating, the aim must be to modify them. Sometimes less harmful preoccupations can be substituted for those that are more inconvenient. A patient who finds it difficult to stop washing his hands or to complete his morning toilet may perhaps be helped to work to a time schedule and to aim at completing a detailed routine within a given time.

It is necessary to discuss with the doctor whether it is more important to reduce anxiety and possibly to allow the patient unlimited time for his compulsive actions, or whether it is better to aim at a workable time schedule which would allow him to continue in gainful employment and to alleviate the resulting anxiety by sedation or other methods. If the latter is the case a careful plan must be worked out and discussed in detail with the patient. He will derive some security from the knowledge that an attempt is being made to establish a workable routine and he will then be better able to tolerate his increased tension.

To be inconsistent, to drive the patient sometimes and at other times to let him take several hours to wash and dress, will increase anxiety and not help him in any way.

(c) *Hysteria*

Although the symptoms manifested in hysteria can be extremely varied the underlying basis is the same. The symptoms serve to solve the patient's difficulty and conflicts in a manner acceptable to himself and which may appear to gain him some advantage.

The mechanism by which the symptoms are produced is always unconscious, but sometimes the purpose they serve is obvious to all but the patient, so that the impression may be given that he is malingering.

Hysterical symptoms may take the form of any physical disorder of those parts of the body which can normally be consciously controlled. They depend to a large extent on the patient's knowledge and conception of physical disorder, but also on the particular stresses from which he needs to escape.

Motor symptoms include paralysis of the limbs, twitchings, tics, fits and aphonia. Sensory symptoms include numbness, anaesthesia, pains, blindness or deafness. Careful neurological examination reveals discrepancies between the distribution of the symptoms and that which would occur if there were an organic basis. The symptoms complained of correspond rather to the patient's own idea of anatomical structure. Such symptoms are referred to as 'conversion symptoms'.

Although the symptoms may be exceedingly incapacitating and his description of them is often highly dramatic, the patient appears fairly complacent about his illness. This is possible because the symptom in fact represents the way in which he has solved an otherwise insoluble problem. He cannot give up the symptom without becoming overwhelmed by difficulties.

Sometimes the patient, instead of finding an escape in physical symptoms, forgets about his problems and behaves as if they did not exist. He may disclaim any knowledge of unpleasant and unacceptable events and suffer from amnesia for a considerable part of his life.

The most spectacular form of dissociation occurs in the type of dual personality illustrated by Robert Louis Stevenson's *Dr Jekyll and Mr. Hyde*, a condition which is very rare.

Symptoms often very closely simulate those of organic illness and are at times actually associated with organic disorders. In many neurological conditions symptoms are aggravated during periods of emotional stress. Symptoms may be suggested to the patient during repeated medical examinations. Physical illness may represent a stress situation to which the patient may respond by developing an hysterical illness. The most difficult problems occur when the patient's physical debility is prolonged by an hysterical illness during a time when compensation claims for accidents are outstanding. The term 'compensation neurosis' is applied to this prolongation of physical incapacity.

Treatment of hysteria does not consist in removing the symptom, but in discovering the conflict situation which the symptom is designed to solve and then to help the patient to find a more satisfactory solution to the problem. The patient's illness demonstrates the need to attract interest and sympathy. He must receive the attention, interest and sympathy of the psychiatrist and the nursing staff. It may be possible to demonstrate to the patient that it is not necessary to maintain the symptom for this purpose and that the nurses accept and respect him.

Many nurses, however, find this a particularly difficult task and tend to treat the patient as if he were deliberately trying to deceive. It cannot be over-emphasized that the hysterical patient who is seeking attention and trying to be loved really needs all the love and attention he can get. He needs to feel successful and requires sufficient encouragement to surmount obstacles in a realistic way.

PSYCHOTIC DISORDERS

Psychotic disorders are those mental disorders which, at least in their most severe forms, affect every aspect of the patient's life and are often sufficiently incapacitating to necessitate admission to hospital.

(a) *Manic-depressive psychosis* is a disturbance of mood, in which elated periods alternate with phases of depression. Some patients experience long periods of normal emotional reactions between attacks of mania or depression, others pass gradually from one phase to the other.

In health, people predisposed to manic-depressive disorders are frequently warm, outgoing people, liable to be moody, but gay, cheerful and hearty when the mood is good. The friendliness and warmth of feeling is appreciated by many friends, and they are popular with their colleagues.

The first attack of mania or depression is often precipated by a crisis in the patient's life; further attacks may occur at regular intervals or may only accompany stressful situations.

In *mania* the patient is happy, elated and feels on top of the world. Everything is wonderful in his eyes, he is full of self-confidence, makes plans for great actions and indulges in feverish activity. His speech is so rapid that it is difficult of comprehension, his thoughts appear to follow each other too rapidly to be communicated in words. The patient's movements are large, often graceful. There is constant activity, but inability to concentrate on any particular task. The patient feels constrained and hemmed in, he is hypersensitive to noise, sometimes the feeling of his clothes irritates him sufficiently to cause him to tear them up. He is highly distractible. Any stimulus, a spoken word, a movement or some sound will set off a new train of thought, words or deeds.

Speech does not follow the usual logic. The sound of words is often the cue to association of ideas. Rhyming and punning are common. For a while the patient's happiness is infectious. However, he easily becomes irritable and sometimes aggressive if he is in any way prevented from carrying out his intentions.

There is serious danger to the patient's health. Often it is difficult to persuade him to take adequate nourishment because he rarely takes the time for a substantial meal. His mouth becomes dry and furred as a result of constant talking. He may become seriously dehydrated, excessive energy output not balanced by adequate diet may lead to exhaustion. Injuries and intercurrent infections may occur if proper safeguards are not taken.

Sedation may be essential, but in view of the patient's poor physical condition this may carry its own dangers.

Treatment consists in providing adequate rest and nourishment and protection from danger. The patient's distractibility can be utilized to avoid injury to any member of the staff or the other patients should he become aggressive. But this distractability interferes with rest unless very skilled nursing is provided. The nurse's tone of voice, the deliberate, slow speech, slow movement, monotony of surroundings, subdued lights and absence of noise all help to calm the patient. Sedation and other forms of physical treatment are discussed later.

In acute mania the patient is too disturbed to be nursed with others.

Hypomania

A state of excitement and overactivity which is less severe but more prolonged sometimes occurs; this is called *hypomania*. All the symptoms of mania are present but in a less serious form. Most of the nursing problems are similar to those occurring in the nursing of manic patients, but since the hypomanic patient is able to be nursed in a ward with others, his effect on these must be taken into account. Often the other patients are at first amused by him. His drive and energy makes him a suitable person to choose as a spokesman and to organize activities for the rest. Gradually the fact that he is not always able to carry out his ideas and that he interferes with the others, makes the latter angry and irritable. Kind intentions are looked upon as interferences and he becomes a target of general hostility.

He requires protection from the less well-controlled patients; friction and quarrels should be prevented. The patient may overestimate his strength and some curtailment of his activities may be necessary.

Occasionally the hypomanic state becomes chronic and keeps the patient in hospital for years. Among the chronic psychiatric hospital patients the hypomanic patient stands out because his drive and his interest in all that is happening are strangely in contrast with the apathy of many of the others. In dress the hypomanic patient is outstanding. He uses every scrap of colourful material to adorn himself. He is the one who comes forward to welcome visitors and to give all the information.

(b) Depression

Depressive reactions often occur alternately with manic episodes. Some patients show recurrent depressive phases during which they require treatment and care. Between these attacks they feel very well indeed but never to the extent of developing a manic reaction.

The depressed patient often feels and looks sad. His movements and thoughts are slow, he stoops, or sits with his head bent low. He does not wish to converse and says as little as possible, slowly and in monosyllables. He is uninterested in his surroundings, unobservant of all but the most depressing events. His thoughts, if he reveals them, centre on unpleasant topics. Guilt and sin are commonly mentioned. The patient considers himself to be wicked, feels that he has committed unforgivable sins and that he deserves to be punished. He may hear voices which accuse him or comment on his unworthiness. His pessimistic concern with his wickedness or his poverty may be held with the force of a delusion.

Some patients suffering from depression do not look sad. Their apparently smiling expression may cause a profound underlying suffering to go unnoticed. In extreme forms of depression the patient does not feel depressed or sad. He may say that he lacks feeling altogether or feels empty. He may have feelings of unreality, the world may seem to have changed, or he himself may feel that he no longer exists or that parts of him have died away.

Loss of appetite, constipation and often nausea, may give rise to delusions, in keeping with the depressive feeling, of having no intestines, of the intestines being eaten away, or of suffering from an incurable disease. He may sleep badly, particularly in the early hours of the morning. There is considerable danger of malnutrition occurring. Lack of interest in personal hygiene or personal appearance may lead to infection. Above all there is the danger of suicide.

Depressive illness of a different kind may occur in people of late middle age. In women the onset of the illness may roughly coincide with the menopause and the term *'involutional melancholia'* is sometimes used to distinguish this disorder from depression occurring in manic-depressive cycles.

Involutional melancholia occurs in people who have never suffered from a depressive illness before, and have not been subject to fluctuating moods. On the contrary, there is often evidence of exceptionally stable temperament, and occasional irritability may have been the only emotional disturbance noticed by the patient or his relatives. The patient may have held the same job for many years, and may be conspicuous for his conscientiousness, reliability and perseverance.

The illness is possibly related to some physiological changes which take place in late middle age, and often an awareness of physiological disturbance is one of its cardinal features. There is very marked anxiety and preoccupation with bodily function. Worry is expressed about bowels, flatulence, indigestion, or about palpitation, flushing, giddiness and blood pressure. Some patients, in the depth of despair, attribute anxiety and depression to physical ill-health and contemplate suicide because of their intolerable fear of chronic disease. In some patients preoccupation with bodily function takes on a delusional character. Such a patient may be convinced that he smells, that his illness is contagious, that he is a danger to others or that his physical debility is the result of divine punishment, or caused by the wickedness of men. Sometimes the illness may be related to changes in the routine of life which had become indispensable for the patient's sense of security. Retirement, loss of a job after some unavoidable absence may precipitate the onset of the depression. Others react to the death of a close friend or relative by becoming depressed. Some women, when they realize that the childbearing period is approaching an end, that the children have grown up and are no longer dependent, feel overwhelmed with a sense of futility and loneliness.

Involutional depression differs from other depressive illnesses in that there is very marked agitation and anxiety but no retardation. The patient feels miserable, hopeless and desperate. The risk of suicide is very great, because the patient has the necessary energy and determination to put plans into action.

The patient's thought content is very similar to that of other depressed patients, but he speaks more, sometimes very rapidly, although he may only repeat incessantly some expression of despair, e.g. 'Dear, oh dear', or he may utter supplications to God for help.

Involutional depression responds particularly favourably to electroconvulsive therapy, although even without this, most patients recover after some months. In manic states and in all forms of depression drug treatment is often found to be effective. During the illness constant vigilance is required to protect the patient from suicidal acts. He requires help to go through a period of intense suffering. The nurse's attitude of sympathy, but unshakable hopefulness, her indication that the patient's life is important, her understanding of the conflict may provide the necessary support during the illness.

(c) Schizophrenic Reactions

Schizophrenia is a term used to describe a variety of disorders with certain characteristics in common but with considerable variations in other respects.

The characteristics found in most schizophrenic patients are a withdrawal of interest from everyday affairs and an emotional coldness.

There is almost certainly a hereditary basis for schizophrenic disorders, but the onset of observable symptoms frequently coincides with some period of emotional stress. There is a relatively high incidence oi mental disorder among relatives of schizophrenic patients. The history of many patients reveals some traumatic incidents during earliest childhood. It may be found that the patient during his earliest years has failed to receive or show the amount of affection considered necessary for normal development, and that his parents appeared disinclined or unable to provide emotional warmth. It is not clear to what extent the patient's emotional detachment is an inherited characteristic and whether the lack of emotional responsiveness was caused by the mother's coldness or the child's own inability to show affection.

When the history of a schizophrenic patient is taken the onset of the illness is usually put down to a specific event in his life. Closer inquiry, however, reveals an insidious onset of the symptoms, and friends and relatives usually agree that over a long period they had observed increasingly strange behaviour on the part of the patient. He has probably very gradually become more aloof, less interested in other people or in events which interest others. He may have spent less and less time with people, and more by himself. His work may have deteriorated over a period of time.

Other symptoms, and the further course of events, vary very greatly, but a number of patterns tend to recur.

Simple Schizophrenic Disorders

These run a progressive course without any highlights. The patient becomes increasingly solitary, more and more detached, unable to show emotional response even to highly significant situations such as the death of a close relative. He appears to be preoccupied with thoughts and ideas which he is unable adequately to communicate to others. His conversation becomes more and more difficult to follow.

Eventually the patient may withdraw entirely from society, cease to go to work, remain in his room and neglect his appearance. His physical health may suffer as a result of lack of exercise and adequate nourishment.

Some patients are eventually admitted to hospital, either when their physical health has deteriorated to such an extent that hospitalization becomes inevitable, or when complaints are made by neighbours, landladies or welfare agencies about neglect, dirt or unacceptable behaviour. Many patients, however, manage to maintain just sufficient interest in personal health and appearance to continue living in the community—alone, friendless, and on a very low economic level. They perform unskilled work, often well below their original capacity, drift from job to job, throw up work without adequate reason, live by themselves in relative squalor and discomfort, or become harmless tramps and vagrants.

Hebephrenic Schizophrenia

This is a highly dramatic disorder coming closest to the popular idea of 'madness'. Often, after a period of insidious withdrawal, the patient enters a phase of wild excitement during which he shows a multitude of florid symptoms of mental disorder. Hallucinations are very common. Voices may be heard accusing the patient of misdeeds, using obscene language or commenting in unflattering terms on his every action. Sometimes the voices give orders, or pronounce prophecies. They may be so authoritative and clear that the patient unquestioningly obeys their commands and performs actions which he considers to be quite alien to his nature. He may attribute the voices to 'God' or to 'the Devil', or may endeavour to find the 'people' who are speaking to him. If he realizes that there is no one present he tends to blame 'wireless' or 'electricity' for the voices.

Difficulties may arise because the voices command the patient to perform antisocial actions, e.g. attacks on others, or may suggest that people harbour evil intentions. The patient may refuse to eat and become completely incapable of continuing any normal activity as a result of his preoccupation with his hallucinatory experiences. Some patients become totally inaccessible, unable to follow ordinary conversation, uninterested in other people's ideas and preoccupied with bizarre thoughts of their own, which they may or may not be able to express. Some are able to give verbal accounts of their thoughts, ascribing significance to events which other people look upon in entirely different perspective. Thoughts do not follow each other in the normal manner and connections appear illogical and bizarre. Often new words are used in an endeavour to communicate highly complicated ideas.

Some patients find it difficult to express their ideas in words. Blocking may occur, the patient suddenly stops, forgets completely what he was saying and continues by discussing an apparently unrelated idea. Methods of expression other than words may be more congenial to the patient. Painting, needlework or modelling often reveal the bizarre nature of his ideas. If he is unoccupied he may laugh and sing loudly, dance, posture and grimace. Laughter and tears follow each other in rapid succession without any apparent cause.

Patients may describe the most bizarre delusions, embodying the latest information about bombs, atomic energy, space travel and telepathy. These are often coloured by personal prejudices, as, for example, those concerning Negroes, Germans or Jews. Very often the patient feels that his chaotic thoughts are not his own, that they have been put into his head and that he is being influenced by evil powers. He perceives everything that is going on around him as being related to himself and interprets everything he sees or hears as an ominous signal passed between people or powers directing his life. Incongruity between feelings and thoughts is often a prominent symptom. The patient professes love for a person he attacks, he may hear of sad news and laugh about it, or may giggle while he himself announces some terrible disaster or recounts a tale of dreadful events.

The episode of acute disturbance is usually short. Hallucinations may occur on a single occasion only, delusions may be fleeting. However, the emotional flattening may persist and the patient may feel bewildered and perplexed.

With or without treatment the patient may recover sufficiently to resume normal life, although probably not quite as fully as formerly.

Relapses are likely to occur, each attack leaving the

patient less well than the previous one, until finally he withdraws from reality and lives in a world of phantasy.

Catatonic Schizophrenia

This condition occurs later in life than the simple or hebephrenic forms of the disorder. Prognosis is somewhat better than for simple or hebephrenic schizophrenia, especially if the patient's prepsychotic personality was mature and well integrated.

The extreme forms of catatonic behaviour are stupor and excitement. The transition from one to the other may be very sudden, and occur almost without forewarning. In complete stupor the patient remains motionless in bed, apparently unaware of what is going on around him. That this has not been the case is sometimes revealed by the patient during a more active phase of his illness, or on recovery. During the stuporosed phase the patient looks perplexed. Eye movements are absent. He is rigid. His position in bed is unusual and does not appear comfortable, although he may resist any attempt to change it. On the other hand, he may quite passively allow his position to be altered. Even if the attitude is abnormal he may maintain it for many hours. This condition is termed 'waxy flexibility' because it feels as if the patient could be moulded into position. Some patients are known to have held their heads a few inches above the pillow for many hours or to have remained standing on one leg until moved by a nurse.

Catatonic patients are said to be negativistic, e.g. remaining mute if asked a question and answering when the questioner passes on to something else, or keeping the mouth tightly closed when an attempt at feeding is made, yet appearing to want the food as soon as it is taken away.

Sometimes quite complex arm movements or body movements are repeated over and over again, but they may be simple in long-standing illness and become barely recognizable gestures.

Stupor may suddenly pass into an outburst of wild excitement, during which violent, aggressive actions may be performed.

It is difficult to establish contact with the patient, and attempts to distract him usually fail. His actions appear to be as incoherent as his words, and at times seem related to hallucinatory commands. He may talk very rapidly. His speech may contain many neologisms, many repetitions, many words but few ideas. If he endeavours to express himself in writing, his disordered thinking becomes evident in the way words are disconnected or distorted, and sentences are not completed. Paper is used in an unusual way. Instead of covering one line after another, starting from the top, a beginning will be made anywhere on the page, and jumping from one part of the sheet to another. Often the paper is used a second time, the patient writing over or between the lines already used until every bit of available space is filled up.

Catatonia often lasts for many years in less acute forms. The patient may show characteristic physical signs, e.g. blue and cold limbs, low pulse rate, low blood pressure, greasy skin, low bodyweight.

Paranoid Schizophrenia

This type of schizophrenic disorder shows the most regular pattern of development. It begins with delusions of a fairly coherent nature. In paranoid schizophrenia it is usually conceivable that the delusional idea expressed by the patient might be true, unlike those of hebephrenic patients, which are so bizarre that they could not possibly be true.

If it is assumed that the patient acts as if his delusional ideas were true, his actions become meaningful and it can be understood why the patient elaborates and enlarges on them and develops resentment against the people around him, whom he considers hostile because they disbelieve his ideas.

Many patients experience hallucinations which they try to explain and to integrate with the delusional ideas, so that one vast delusional system is developed which may persist for years and continue to grow. Some, however, become perplexed by their own feelings and thoughts which they may recognize as strange and, therefore, attribute to the influence of outside forces. Various delusional ideas, instead of becoming systematized may be fleeting only, changing from day to day. The patient's emotional state depends largely on his delusions, varying from abject misery to states of overwhelming happiness and ecstasy, and on the extent to which he continues to be distressed by the presumed hostility of the world around him.

In chronic paranoid illness the patient may appear able to adapt himself to some situation in which he feels safe and protected from the evil influences of those he fears. He may appear to be quite normal so long as no major changes occur in his life. Alternatively, the patient may appear well in a new environment if he feels he has escaped from his persecutors. Gradually, however, his new environment is drawn into the delusional system and only another move will satisfy the patient.

The prognosis in schizophrenic disorders is less favourable than in other forms of disorder. Many patients, however, recover from their more acute schizophrenic attack and remain apparently well for some time. Further attacks may last longer and leave the patient less well, until finally deterioration becomes so disabling that hospitalization for chronicity may be necessary.

Physical treatment and good nursing care shorten attacks, make recovery more complete and, even in the case of the permanently hospitalized patient, increase the patient's happiness and usefulness.

One of the nurse's most important functions is to establish and maintain emotional rapport with the patient and to prevent the emotional isolation which occurs in schizophrenic patients. Many nursing problems arise as a result of the patient's delusions. Refusal of food, episodic outbursts of violence, and incontinence are some of the difficulties, and these are dealt with in earlier chapters.

Appendix

Notes on the Mental Health Act 1959
and the Mental Health (Scotland) Act 1960

The main principles on which the Acts are based are:

1. That patients suffering from mental disorder should as far as possible be treated in or outside hospital on the same basis as patients suffering from any other disorder. They should be able to enter *any hospital capable of offering treatment.* They should enter hospital or leave hospital with no more formality or restrictions than any other patients.
2. That, outside hospital, provisions should be made for treatment and care comparable to those offered to people suffering from other disorders.
3. That hospitals which offer psychiatric treatment should be free to refuse admission if they feel unable to help the patient or for any other reason just as other hospitals are.
4. That the provisions made for the fairly small number of patients who must be detained against their will should entail only a minimal amount of legal restriction.

In order to achieve these objects, *all* previous legislation relating both to *Mental Illness* and what was formerly known as *Mental Deficiency* is repealed. *One* Act has replaced all former legislation and it covers disorders not formerly dealt with.

The term *Mental Disorder* is used to cover all disorders which are dealt with under the Act. The definition in the Act of 'Mental Disorder' is: 'Mental illness, arrested or incomplete development, psychopathic disorder and any other disorder or disability of mind'.

There are four subdivisions of Mental Disorder recognized for the purposes of the compulsory provisions of the act of 1959:

1. Mental illness
2. Severe subnormality
3. Subnormality
4. Psychopathic disorder.

The definition of Subnormality includes a statement that it is 'a state of arrested or incomplete development of mind, and that the patient requires or is susceptible to medical treatment or other special care or training'.

The definition of Psychopathic disorder is as follows: 'A persistent disorder or disability of mind (whether or not including subnormality of intelligence) which results in abnormally aggressive or seriously irresponsible conduct on the part of the patient and requires or is susceptible to medical treatment'.

The Scottish act does not define the categories. The term 'Mental Disorder' means Mental Illness and Mental Defect. The latter term remains in use and no definition of Psychopathic Disorder is included in the Act.

Admission Without Compulsion

Patients in all four of these categories can be admitted to any hospital without compulsion or application. It is not necessary that the patient should be capable of expressing a wish to be admitted. As long as he is not actively unwilling to enter hospital his admission can be informal.

In the case of patients suffering from mental illness, informal admission is nearly always possible because patients are either too ill to object or quite readily agree to enter hospital.

Most patients suffering from severe subnormality can be informally admitted as they are incapable of expressing any objection and are, by definition, incapable of living an independent life.

Compulsory Admission

Some patients suffering from mental illness, subnormality or psychopathic disorder may have to be compulsorily admitted to hospital. Patients in the two categories of (i) Subnormality (ii) Psychopathic disorder, can be compulsorily admitted only if they are under 21 years and they cannot be detained beyond the age of 25 years except in special circumstances. Compulsory admission occurs on *application* from the nearest relatives or from a *mental welfare officer* (mental health officers in Scotland).

Some relevant sections of the 1959 Act dealing with compulsory detention are:

Section 29. In emergency, application from the relative or Mental Welfare Officer need only be supported by *one* medical certificate. Within 72 hours the recommendation ceases to have effect unless a second medical certificate is issued. (In Scotland emergency admission is for seven days).

Section 25. In ordinary circumstances or within 72 hours after admission, under Section 29, the patient is admitted for *observation*. This requires an application from the relative or Mental Welfare Officer and two medical recommendations. The patient may be detained for up to 28 days. (No provisions exist in the Scottish Act for admission for observation.)

Section 26. Should it still be necessary the patient can be compulsorily detained for *treatment*.

The two medical recommendations must:

(a) Give a clinical description of the patient's mental condition.

(b) State the form of mental disorder from which he is suffering and state that it is of a nature and degree which warrants detention in hospital for medical treatment.

(c) Indicate whether other methods of care are available and if so why they are not appropriate and why informal admission is not suitable.

A patient admitted for treatment may be detained for one year in the first instance. If it is considered that a further period is necessary in the interest of the patient's health, safety or for the protection of others, the authority to detain the patient can be renewed for one year and after that every two years. (In Scotland authority for detention of a patient still requires approval of the Sheriff. The patient has the right to appeal to the Sheriff against his detention.)

Patients who feel that they are wrongfully detained may apply to a *Mental Health Review Tribunal* for a review, within six months from the date of admission and again within six months of every renewal of the compulsory detention order. (In Scotland there is the Mental Welfare Commission, consisting of seven to nine commissioners whose duty it is to exercise protective functions on behalf of the patient.)

If a mentally disordered person is convicted of an offence the Court may order the patient to be compulsorily admitted to hospital.

The patient's nearest relative has the power to order *the discharge* of a patient who is compulsorily detained under Section 26.

Only if the patient is likely to act dangerously can the medical officer refuse discharge. If the patient is ordered to be admitted by a Court the relatives cannot ask for the patient's discharge.

Students who are interested in details of the Mental Treatment Act are advised to consult the Act itself or the National Association of Mental Health's Guide to the Mental Health Act. The Act for Scotland (1960) and N. Ireland (1961) differ slightly from the Act for England and Wales.

Glossary

———

I AM *indebted to the late Editor of the Royal Medico-Psychological Association's* Handbook for Psychiatric Nurses *for permission to use extracts from the glossary in the Handbook.*

This glossary is intended to supplement the main text by providing an explanation, as well as a definition, of certain important terms. Some common terms are not included because they are adequately explained in the text. Terms used in organic medicine have generally not been included, and for definitions and explanations of these a general nursing dictionary should be consulted.

Acting Out. Attempts by some patients undergoing psychotherapy to reduce their emotional discomfort by releasing their feelings in disturbed behaviour. The latter is unconsciously determined and reflects previous unresolved conflicts and attitudes towards important figures during childhood. Such behaviour is consequently often aggressive and anti-social, but it is unsatisfactory to apply the term, as is sometimes done, to all disturbed behaviour shown by patients with neurotic or personality disorders.

The aim of treatment is often to help the patient to talk about his difficulties (to verbalize) instead of acting out.

Affect. Emotion, feeling or mood. Disturbances of affect of various kinds may occur in psychiatric disorders (for example, lability of mood, cyclothymia, flattening, incongruity and inappropriateness of affect).

Affective Disorders. Psychiatric disorders in which the chief feature is a relatively prolonged affective change of abnormal degree, i.e. depression or mania.

Ambivalence. The existence, at the same time, of contradictory emotional feelings towards an object, commonly of love and hate for another person. Some ambivalence is a normal phenomenon in interpersonal relationships, but when it occurs to a marked degree it may lead to internal conflict and symptoms of psychological disturbance.

Amnesia. A loss or absence of memory which may cover a variable period of time in the recent or remote past, and may be complete or partial (patchy).

Disturbance of memory is most commonly found in association with intellectual impairment as a symptom of dementia resulting from organic brain disease or degeneration. In such cases memory for recent events is lost first, but the impairment may later extend progressively back into the past and even into childhood. In the so-called ' amnestic ' (Korsakoff's) syndrome, however, it is the complete inability to remember current events and the fact that the patient invents stories to fill in the gap (confabulation) that is the most striking feature, and there may be little or no evidence of any other intellectual deficit.

The first stage in the process of remembering is registration of the material to be subsequently recalled, and it is evident that this may be disturbed in states of impaired concentration. This may occur in functional psychotic disorders so that memory may be patchy for events during the acute stage of the illness. In the same way, a partial amnesia may be left after states of clouded consciousness and there is obviously a complete amnesia covering any period of unconsciousness.

The amnesia following head injury may however cover

a period that exceeds the duration of unconsciousness. The loss of memory for events prior to the injury is spoken of as retrograde or pre-traumatic amnesia. The anterograde or post-traumatic amnesia extends from time of injury until continuous awareness by the patient. There may be some patchy memories towards the end of this period owing to the stage of clouded consciousness through which the patient passes before full consciousness is regained.

Amnesia may also occur as a hysterical phenomenon, sometimes associated with a fugue state. In such cases it often covers a long period, perhaps of many years, and there may be a discrepancy between the patient's ability to perform learned activities, or the knowledge he displays, and the extent of his amnesia.

Aphasia. The loss of the ability to express meaning by the use of speech or writing, or to understand spoken or written language, the former being described as motor and the latter as sensory aphasia. A lesser degree of impairment is known as dysphasia. Different types of aphasia arise from injury, disease or degeneration of various brain centres.

Aphonia. Loss of voice. May occur as a hysterical phenomenon.

Ataxia. Loss or impairment of muscular co-ordination, resulting in an inability to perform accurate voluntary movement. In the upper limbs this is manifest as a clumsiness in handling and manipulating objects, and in the lower limbs as an unsteady or staggering gait. Ataxia may arise from injury, disease or degeneration of the brain or spinal cord, from toxic conditions or may be hysterical in origin.

Compulsion. A term restricted by some psychiatrists to an obsessional act, but used by others for all obsessional symptoms, i.e. compulsive words, phrases, ideas, thoughts, images and fears, as well as impulses. Compulsive actions are recognized by the patient to be morbid and irrational, and he struggles against them. Resistance is, however, usually associated with mounting anxiety which is relieved once the action is performed.

Conditioning. The process, described by Pavlov, by which a new stimulus, known as the ' conditioned ' stimulus, comes to produce a response which is normally the result of another stimulus, the ' unconditioned ' stimulus. Thus, in the classical experiment which he performed with the dog, Pavlov found that the repeated association of food (the unconditioned stimulus) with the sound of a bell, eventually led to the response of salivation being elicited by the bell alone (the conditioned stimulus).

In a similar way, the response of fear, which normally occurs in situations of danger, may become conditioned to various stimuli which are not in themselves usually fear-provoking, through some association with such a situation. Thus a pilot may acquire a phobia for flying following an air crash, or a child may become terrified of all dogs after being attacked by one.

It is uncertain to what extent such conditioning may contribute to the causes of phobic and some other psychiatric disorders, but techniques for deconditioning (removal of conditioning) are being used with some success in the treatment of selected cases of phobic anxiety. Conversely, the process of conditioning an unpleasant response, such as vomiting, to the hitherto pleasant stimulus of alcohol is used in the ' aversion ' treatment of alcoholism.

Delusion. A false belief which, in the face of contrary evidence, is held with conviction and is unmodifiable by appeals to reason or logic that would be acceptable to other persons of the same religious or cultural background.

A delusion signifies a break with reality which justifies its description as a psychotic symptom, and ome psychiatrists would further hold that any condition in which it is found should be considered a psychosis. Beyond this however, the mere presence of a delusion is not diagnostic of any particular psychiatric disorder, though some types of delusion may be characteristic of certain conditions.

Delusions may be classified by (a) mode of origin (b) content, and (c) degree of systematization.

(a) By mode of origin a distinction can be made between ' primary ' and ' secondary ' delusions. Primary or autochthonous delusions appear suddenly, fully developed and without warning, and are practically diagnostic of schizophrenia. By contrast, secondary or interpretative delusions may occur in most psychotic disorders, and arise as a response of the patient to other symptoms of the illness. Thus, for example, delusions of guilt and unworthiness may arise in the setting of the depressive mood in involutional melancholia, or delusions of persecution in schizophrenia when auditory hallucinations are attributed to a hostile person or organization.

(b) In terms of their content several types of delusion are recognized. Delusions of grandeur may occur in G.P.I., mania and schizophrenia. As the name implies, these are false beliefs concerning the patient's status and power. Paranoid is the term used to describe all delusions of being affected in some harmful or persecutory way. These may occur not only in schizophrenia and the paranoid states, but also in affective disorders, organic syndromes, and alcoholic and drug psychoses. In depressive illness, however, the patient will commonly accept such persecution as his just due, in keeping with his feeling of guilt and self-reproach. Delusions of reference are common in schizophrenia, but may also occur in affective illness and sometimes as a reaction in abnormally sensitive personalities. The patient believes that people, things and events refer to him in a special way. Thus people, even complete strangers in the street, look at him and he knows they are talking about him, or items on the radio and in the newspaper are really referring to him. Delusions of influence are often secondary to the disturbances of thought, perception and volition, which occur in schizophrenia. The patient complains that his thoughts, feelings and actions are influenced and controlled by some outside agency via radio waves, hypnotism and telepathy. These are also sometimes referred to as passivity feelings. Delusions of self-reproach, guilt and unworthiness are found in depressive illness and are in keeping with the prevailing mood of the patient. He reproaches himself for past failures and misdeeds which are often of a trivial nature. In involutional melancholia such delusions may become quite extravagant so that, for example, disasters and catastrophes in the world are held to be the result of the patient's sins. Hypochondriacal delusions are common in depressions of later life. A frequent complaint is of blockage of the bowels, and other beliefs include the presence of venereal disease and cancer. Somatic delusions may arise from unusual bodily sensations in schizophrenia. They are frequently bizarre, the patient believing for example that his appearance has completely changed and that he is turning into a woman. Nihilistic delusions typically occur in involutional melancholia. The patient believes that he is destroyed in part or totally, so that, for example, his inside has rotted away, or he is already dead and in hell.

(c) The degree of logical relationship between delusions may vary. At one extreme, patients to whom the diagnosis ' paranoia ' is sometimes given may gradually develop, step by step, a system of delusions that is constructed in a logical manner and based on a single original false belief. Such delusions are said to be systematized. At the other extreme, delusions in delirium are commonly short-lived, changeable and unconnected with each other, i.e. unsystematized. Between these two extremes any degree of connection can occur between co-existent delusions.

Depersonalization. A state in which the individual experiences a change in himself as a loss of his own identity or reality. It is characteristically very difficult to describe directly; the patient may use terms like odd, strange or peculiar, or expressions such as ' like an automaton ' and ' as if in a dream ' or may speak of feeling ' unreal '. Sometimes included under the term depersonalization is the comparable state of derealization in which it is the outer world that appears changed or unreal, rather than the individual himself. Again, this may be described in various ways, e.g. ' everything seems flat ', ' as if the world is on the other side of a pane of glass '. Both states may be found in association, or either may occur alone.

Mild, transient depersonalization is a not uncommon occurrence in normal individuals, usually when fatigued. In a more severe form it can be a feature of most psychiatric disorders, and may simply represent the patient's way of interpreting changes in himself brought about by the illness.

It should be noted that in depersonalization the individual or the world is not described as actually changes, but 'as if' it is. A belief in an actual change may occur at times, but then denotes a delusional development.

Disorientation. Disturbance of the individual's appreciation of his position in time or space, or of his own identity, found in states of impaired consciousness, and revealed in his answers to questions concerning his identity, as to where he thinks he is, or what he believes to be the time, day of the week, or date.

Empathy. In psychiatric usage, the degree to which the observer is able to enter into the thoughts and feelings of the patient and establish good contact.

Endogenous and Exogenous. Endogenous—originating from within. Exogenous—originating from outside. Used in psychiatry to distinguish between those cases of depressive illness which cannot easily be explained as a response to the patient's external circumstances and which are therefore assumed to be due to an innate predisposition to such illness (endogenous), and those which appear to be entirely related to the patient's situation (exogenous or reactive) (See also *Reactive*). Some psychiatrists hold that it is generally possible to allot cases of depressive illness to one or other of these two categories. Others, however, are of the opinion that this is only possible in a few cases which represent extreme examples, and that most depressions show evidence of both endogenous and exogenous factors.

Fugue. A state of altered awareness during which an individual suddenly forgets part or the whole of his life, leaves his home and wanders away. He often travels some distance until, just as suddenly, he becomes aware again of his identity. The place where he finds himself may be strange to him, but not infrequently it is somewhere that was of emotional importance at some earlier period in his life. He is likely to have, for a time at least, a complete amnesia for the period of the wandering or fugue itself.

The fugue is commonly a hysterical phenomenon, serving as a means of escape from some unpleasant situation or return to a place which was associated with a happier period in the patient's life which he (unconsciously) wishes to relive. Fugues may also occur occasionally in depressive illness, schizophrenia and epilepsy.

Hallucination. A false sensory perception which arises on its own, in the absence of a corresponding objective stimulus. Any form of sensation may be involved, so that in simple terms a hallucination can mean seeing, hearing, smelling, tasting or feeling something that is not actually present.

A hallucination should be distinguished from an illusion, another disorder of perception, i.e. mistaking something that is seen or heard for something else.

Hallucinations may be experienced by some normal individuals between the sleeping and waking state, i.e. just before going off to sleep or before fully awakening, and these are termed hypnagogic. In general, however, hallucinations are only found in mental disorder and are regarded as a psychotic symptom. Particular types of hallucination may be characteristic of some psychiatric disorders, or rarely found in others.

Visual hallucinations (i.e. of sight) usually occur in states of altered consciousness and should always suggest the possibility of an organic condition. In delirium and toxic confusional states, visual hallucinations are more common than auditory, and characteristically take the form of people, animals or scenes which are well-defined, detailed and frequently terrifying. Hallucinations in an epileptic aura are often visual and may be of a simple undifferentiated kind such as balls of fire, or more complex with scenes of elaborate detail. In epileptic twilight states visual hallucinations are characteristically vivid, with complex scenes that are frequently coloured and moving. Visual hallucinations are rare in schizophrenia but may occur in the acute early stages of the illness, sometimes with some disturbance of consciousness. Visual hallucinations do not occur in depressive illnesses. Visual hallucinations very occasionally occur as a hysterical manifestation and the images which appear have a psychological significance to the patient, e.g. a dead parent or a religious figure.

Auditory hallucinations (i.e. of hearing) occur most frequently in schizophrenia but are also found less commonly in certain other psychiatric conditions, particularly in states of impaired consciousness. In delirium they tend to be of a simple undifferentiated kind such as buzzing or ringing, but threatening voices may occur in the subacute delirious states. The predominant symptom in alcoholic hallucinosis is auditory hallucination, which initially is unformed, but gradually becomes differentiated into voices. Auditory hallucinations in an epileptic aura are usually unformed, but epileptic patients suffering from dreamy states or chronic paranoid hallucinatory states commonly hear voices that are accusatory and abusive. Auditory hallucinations may occur in severe depressive disorders and the content is then in keeping with the depressed mood. The patient may hear voices saying that he is an evil person, lives a sinful life and is due for punishment. In schizophrenia auditory hallucinations are a common but not invariable feature. They may occur early or late in the illness, on only one occasion or repeatedly. The voices may be recognizable or not, distinct or indistinct, abusive or encouraging. They may describe all that the patient does, repeat aloud his thoughts, threaten or give him commands. They may appear to come from outside the body but are often located within the head and sometimes even other parts of the body such as the chest or abdomen.

Olfactory hallucinations (i.e. of smell) may occur in schizophrenia, a patient claiming, for example, that he can smell gas with which enemies are poisoning him. It is also characteristic for the seizures of temporal lobe epilepsy to commence with an olfactory hallucination.

Gustatory hallucinations (i.e. of taste) occur in the same conditions as those of smell. Thus a patient suffering from schizophrenia may complain of a change in the taste of food which indicates to him that he is being poisoned, and gustatory hallucinations may also occur as the aura of temporal lobe epilepsy.

Tactile hallucinations (i.e. of touch) may be found in states of altered consciousness and schizophrenia. They occur very characteristically in cocaine psychosis, which is a subacute delirious state due to prolonged exposure to the drug and probably arises from its effect on peripheral nerves. Patients complain that there are small animals, such as lice, on the skin and may even see them as visual hallucinations. Tactile hallucinations are not uncommon in schizophrenia and may lead to secondary delusional interpretation by the patient, e.g. that rays are being played upon him. They are often localized to the genital region and may then give rise to delusions of sexual interference.

Illusion. A false perception due to distortion of a real sensory perception. An illusion should be distinguished from a hallucination, which is a primary perception in the absence of objective stimulus. For example, if a patient mistakenly interprets a pattern on a wallpaper as grinning faces or eyes watching him, this is an illusion. If, on the other hand, he sees the figure of a man sitting in an empty chair, it is a hallucination.

Illusions may involve any of the senses, are more common at night, and generally occur in states of altered consciousness. It is not always possible, however, to be certain from a patient's account whether an abnormal perceptual experience is an illusion or a hallucination. This is particularly true in schizophrenia and some affective disorders when, for example, patients describe hostile remarks as having been made by people nearby, or see strange things in their room at night.

Insight. Term having more than one meaning in psychiatric usage, but most commonly applied to the recognition by a patient that he is ill. Insight in this sense may be complete, partial or absent, and may change during the course of an illness. Thus a patient who at the beginning of his illness holds delusions may later, with improvement in his condition, develop insight and realize that they were false beliefs arising out of illness. The presence or absence of insight is sometimes used as a criterion for distinguishing between neurotic and psychotic illness respectively, but the difference is seldom clear-cut. The term is also used in a broader sense to mean the understanding by an individual of the underlying reasons for his feelings, attitudes and behaviour, the achieving of such insight being one of the aims of the more radical types of psychotherapy.

Neurosis. See Psychosis.

Phobia. An excessive or irrational fear of a particular object or situation. Phobias for a very wide range of objects and situations can occur, but those which are found most commonly are sometimes given specific descriptive names, e.g. fear of enclosed places—claustrophobia; of open spaces—agoraphobia. Phobias may occur on their own or in association with other symptoms as part of an anxiety state. In such phobias, anxiety is aroused only by the particular object or situation.

However, the term phobia is also sometimes applied to fears with a compulsive quality which are found in obsessional disorder, e.g. those of contamination. Here, the fear is present in the mind most or all of the time, and has the characteristic features of an obsession, i.e. a subjective sense of compulsion and of internal resistance to it.

Psychodynamic. The understanding and interpretation of psychiatric symptoms or abnormal behaviour in terms of unconscious mental mechanisms, e.g. anxiety as the result of repressed aggression, or obsessional symptoms as a defence against forbidden wishes.

Psychopathology. Term used in various ways but generally applied to the study of psychiatric symptoms and disorders in terms of the psychological processes involved.

Psychosis and Neurosis. The terms ' psychosis ' and ' neurosis ' have been used for many years to separate mental illnesses into two groups corresponding generally to those disorders in which the patient is regarded as being ' out of his mind ', ' insane ' or ' mad '— the psychoses—and the remaining milder ' nervous ' illnesses—the neuroses.

The chief points of difference which are customarily considered in making such a distinction are the following:

1. *Severity*
   Psychosis: Major
   Neurosis: Minor
2. *Nature*
   Psychosis: A disease entity with a supposedly physical basis which is genetically determined.
   Neurosis: A reaction to stressful circumstances in a personality predisposed as a result of adverse experiences in childhood.
3. *Contact with reality*
   Psychosis: Loss of contact, as shown by the presence of delusions and hallucinations.
   Neurosis: Normal contact.
4. *Empathy of observer*
   Psychosis: Lack of empathy felt by observer.
   Neurosis: Observer able to feel empathic ' understanding ' of patient's condition as an exaggeration of normal experience.
5. *Insight*
   Psychosis: Absent
   Neurosis: Present

It must be emphasized, however, that the distinction between psychosis and neurosis is by no means as clear-cut and simple as described above, and in many instances it is difficult to decide in which group to place a particular patient or condition. For example, on the one hand some patients may be quite severely disturbed, yet in other respects show features of a neurosis; while on the other hand patients may hold delusions without acting upon them so that they may, superficially at least, show little evidence of illness at all. Some ' psychotic ' patients may have quite good insight into their condition so that they are well aware of being ill, while some patients with 'neurotic' disorders may show little insight into the nature of their illness. Quite apart from these and other discrepancies between clinical features, it remains unproven that the 'psychoses' are disease entities with a physical basis and differ in this way from the 'neuroses'.

For these reasons, many psychiatrists do not attempt to make a distinction between psychosis and neurosis, but prefer to use a general term such as 'illness' or 'disorder' for all conditions, e.g. manic-depressive disorder, obsessional disorder, instead of manic-depressive psychosis and obsessional neuroses. They may still however describe particular symptoms, e.g. delusions and hallucinations, as 'psychotic' in the sense that they indicate a break with reality, and others, e.g. phobias and obsessions, as 'neurotic'.

Reactive. (See also *Endogenous* and *Exogenous*). Term applied to those cases of depressive illness that are considered to arise as a direct response of the patient to adverse external circumstances. Also referred to as 'exogenous depression'. Sometimes also applied to certain disorders with psychotic features, particularly to some occurring during adolescence.

Sibling. One of two or more offspring of the same mother and father. Thus the brothers and sisters of an individual are spoken of as his 'siblings' or 'sibs' for short. If one of his parents has had children by a previous marriage, then they are his 'half-sibs' because he shares with them a common parent. If either his father or his mother remarries someone who already has children by a previous marriage, then these, who are not blood relatives, are described as his 'step-sibs', because they are the offspring of his step-parent.

Syndrome. A group of symptoms and/or signs that are recognized as frequently occurring together and to which it is therefore convenient to give a label for descriptive purposes.

Index

NOTES

NOTES

NOTES

NOTES

NOTES

NOTES

NURSING BOOKS

New Books

Hull & Isaacs
Do-it-Yourself Revision for Nurses: Books 1 & 2
Do It Yourself Revision is an entirely new concept which provides the student nurse with a systematic and interesting method of revision by which she can study a particular subject, answer questions selected from recent State Final Examinations, and mark her replies against model answers provided.

Book 1   144 pages   4 illus.   50p.   *Books 3 & 4 in preparation*
Book 2   144 pages   7 illus.   50p.

Chisholm
An Insight into Health Visiting
Explains to the student nurse why she needs to learn about health visiting, what she will learn when seconded to the health visitor or district nurse, where she will see the health visitor at work and the difference between hospital and community nursing. *102 pages   60p.*

Miles
Baillière's Handbook of First Aid
The sixth edition of this famous Handbook has been extensively revised by STANLEY MILES. While the comprehensive practical first aid instruction of the original authors, which has given the Handbook its reputation as a complete and authoritative work, has been retained, there has been considerable rewriting of the text to include the technical advances in cardiac and respiratory resuscitation and the treatment of shock and burns which have taken place recently.
6th edn.   352 pages   180 illus.   £1.00

Mountjoy & Wythe
Nursing Care of the Unconscious Patient
This new book has been written to help nurses and others responsible for the care of patients whose level of consciousness is abnormal, for whatever reason and wherever the patient is being nursed.
104 pages   11 illus.   90p.

Meering & Stacey
Nursery Nursing *(A Handbook of Child Care)*
A complete textbook covering the syllabuses for the National Nursery Examination Board and the Examination in Nursery Nursing of the Royal Society of Health. In this new edition the age range covered has been extended to 7 years old.
5th edn.   approx. 400 pages   75 illus.   £2.50

BAILLIÈRE TINDALL   **7 & 8 Henrietta Street
London WC2E 8QE**

Reference Books

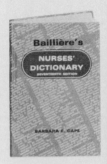
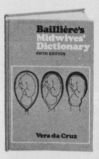
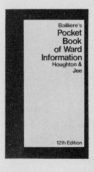

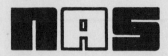

Standard Textbooks

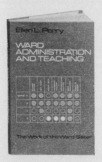

WARD ADMINISTRATION & TEACHING
By Ellen L. Perry

"This is a book which has long been needed. Every trained nurse could learn something from it. While ward sisters put into practice the ideals and ideas outlined, we need have no fears for 'patient care' in our hospitals nor for the practical training of the nurse." *Nursing Mirror*

304 pages   *11 illus.*   *£2.00*

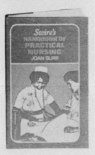

SWIRE'S HANDBOOK OF PRACTICAL NURSING
Revised by Joan Burr

Changes in the syllabus of training have necessitated a major revision for this edition and Miss Burr has taken the opportunity to make many changes of approach to stress the human angle and to enable the nurse to appreciate her surroundings in the hospital and in the community. Care has been taken to cover the syllabus fully, and the use of simple language and illustrated examples ensure the maintained interest of the pupil.

6th Edition
308 pages   *57 illus.*   *£1.00*

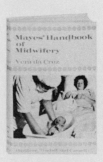

MAYES' HANDBOOK OF MIDWIFERY
Revised by V. Da Cruz

"In this Seventh Edition, Miss da Cruz has incorporated the many new trends and advances made in recent years ... The text is set out with clear headings and good illustrations which make revision easy." *Maternal and Child Care*

458 pages   *156 illus.*   *10 plates*   *£1.80*

BAILLIÈRE TINDALL   7 & 8 Henrietta Street
London WC2E 8QE

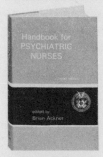

HANDBOOK FOR PSYCHIATRIC NURSES
Edited by the late Brian Ackner

"The R.M.P.A. is to be congratulated on sustaining its great tradition in nursing education by re-modelling its famous 'Handbook' to produce an entirely new account of psychiatry for nurses . . . this is an extremely readable and useful book."
9th Edition   *Nursing Mirror*

364 pages   **1 illus.**   **£2.00**

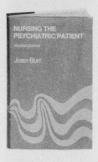

NURSING THE PSYCHIATRIC PATIENT
By Joan Burr

"This book has rapidly been acclaimed as an excellent addition to the psychiatric nursing textbooks already available, and it certainly provides a masterly account of what caring for the mentally ill is about. . . . it is written with such sympathy that, should somebody recognise a description of their own difficulties, they could well gain comfort from the fact that such a helpful understanding is being disseminated."
2nd Edition   *Nursing Times reviewing the first edition*

308 pages   **10 illus.**   **hard cover £1.50**
paperback £1.00

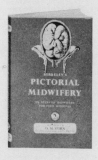

BERKELEY'S PICTORIAL MIDWIFERY
Revised by D. M. Stern

A pictorial survey with excellent illustrations accompanied by clear descriptive text, which will prove invaluable to both the student and qualified midwife alike.

The book has a dual role, providing a text and atlas of theory and a reference for the practical aspects of the subject.

5th Edition

176 pages   **224 illus.**   **2 coloured plates**   **£1.40**

BAILLIÈRE TINDALL
7 & 8 Henrietta Street
London WC2E 8QE

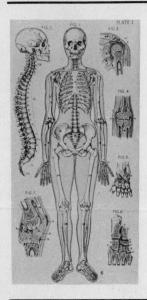